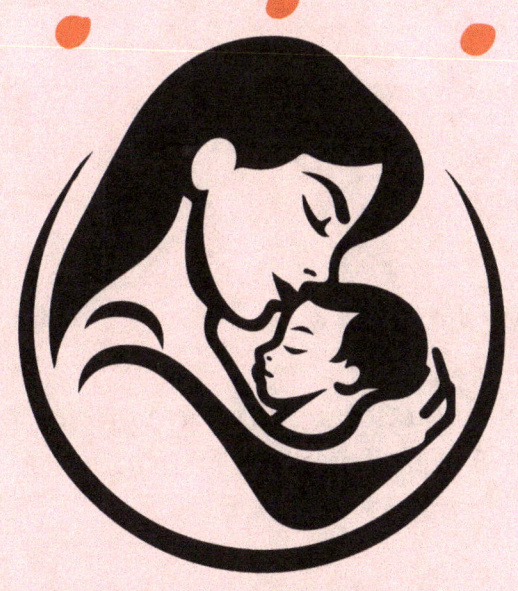

Whispers of Warmth

A Confession from Mother's First Love

By Vicky V. Choudhary

Copyright and Disclaimer

Copyright 2025 @ Vicky V. Choudhary

All rights are reserved. Reproduction of any form or electronic or tangible storage of this work requires express prior authorization from the promoter.

The author wrote this creative emotional inspirational book as if it were an unborn child expressing thoughts to their mother. The book aims to create emotional support for expecting mothers through personal reflections which help build a bond during their pregnancy. The book does not function as a medical guide while providing no professional medical or psychological or health advice. The emotional and poetic contents within this work function solely as written expressions with no purpose of substituting the knowledge of qualified medical providers. Every pregnancy journey is unique. Health-related decision-making should only be guided by medical professionals such as doctors, or licensed specialists. The author and publisher assume no responsibility or liability for any consequence resulting from the use or interpretation of this book's content.

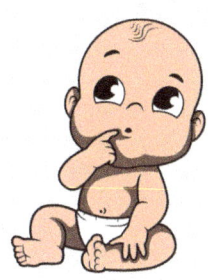

Flow of the Book

- Dedication Page
- Foreword
- Chapter 1: A Bond Begins — 8
- Chapter 2: Growing Together, Stronger Each Day — 14
- Chapter 3: Nurturing Love, Nurturing Life — 20
- Chapter 4: Journeying Through Changes — 26
- Chapter 5: Celebrating Milestones, Cherishing Moments — 32
- Chapter 6: Finding Peace Within — 38
- Chapter 7: Radiating Love and Light — 44
- Chapter 8: Nourishing Body and Soul — 50
- Chapter 9: Embracing the Unknown, Trusting the Journey — 56
- Chapter 10: A Promise of Love — 62
- Closing Note ("Thank you for walking this journey with me.") — 66

Dedication

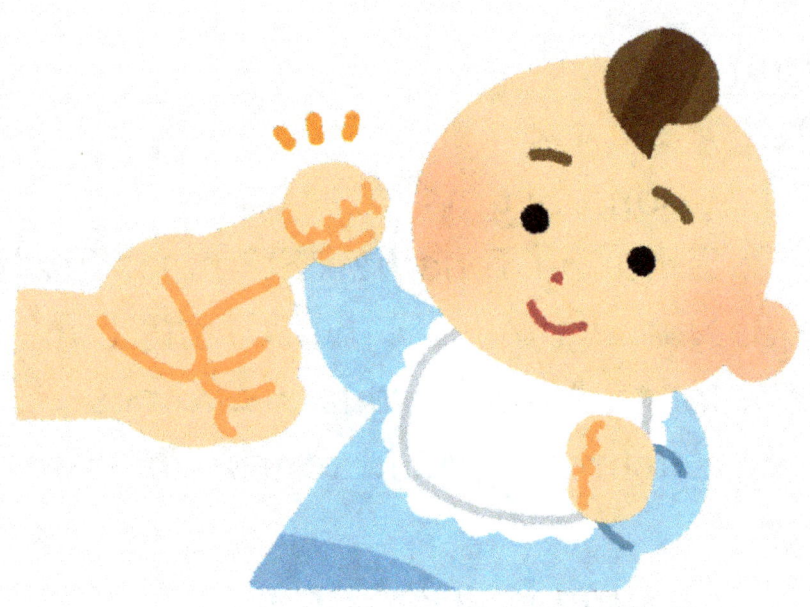

This book is dedicated
to
'Lovely Mothers'

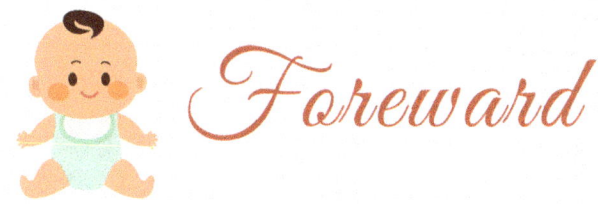

Foreward

Whispers of Warmth is a journey told through the soft, imagined voice of an unborn child to the mother who carries them with love.

Each chapter holds a moment—a heartbeat, a hope, a whisper of connection growing stronger with every passing day. Within these pages, you'll find the invisible thread that ties you to your baby, long before the first cry, the first cuddle, or the first hello.

This is a story written not in ink but in feeling.

In the hush of midnight thoughts, in the flutter of tiny kicks, in the quiet spaces where love speaks loudest without words.

May these whispers wrap gently around your heart. May they bring you comfort, joy, and a deep knowing that you are never alone on this journey.

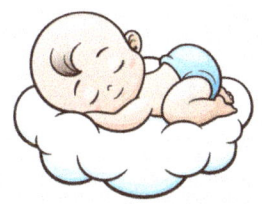

Before We Start

"The Path lies beneath the Eyes of Wisdom,
Roar comes from the courageous heart,
Kindness lies in the helping hands,
Charm lies in the smiling face,
Internal peace lies in your calm mind,
Love dwells in the Pure Soul &
The righteousness lies in following these principles."

My lovely reader,
This is one of my poems that is closest to my heart. Though written by me, it is showcased by all the lovely people I have met in my life.
Wishing You-
Happy Whispers of Warmth!!
Happy reading! Enjoy your book!

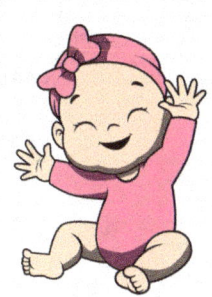

Chapter 1
A Bond Begins

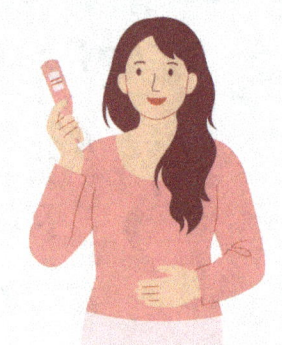

The tender beginning
of an everlasting bond

Whispers from Your Baby

"When did you first recognize my presence at that specific moment? The feelings you experienced deserve your words. Show the amazement along with the happiness and minor concerns. The initial feelings between us have been embedded into our relationship from the beginning."

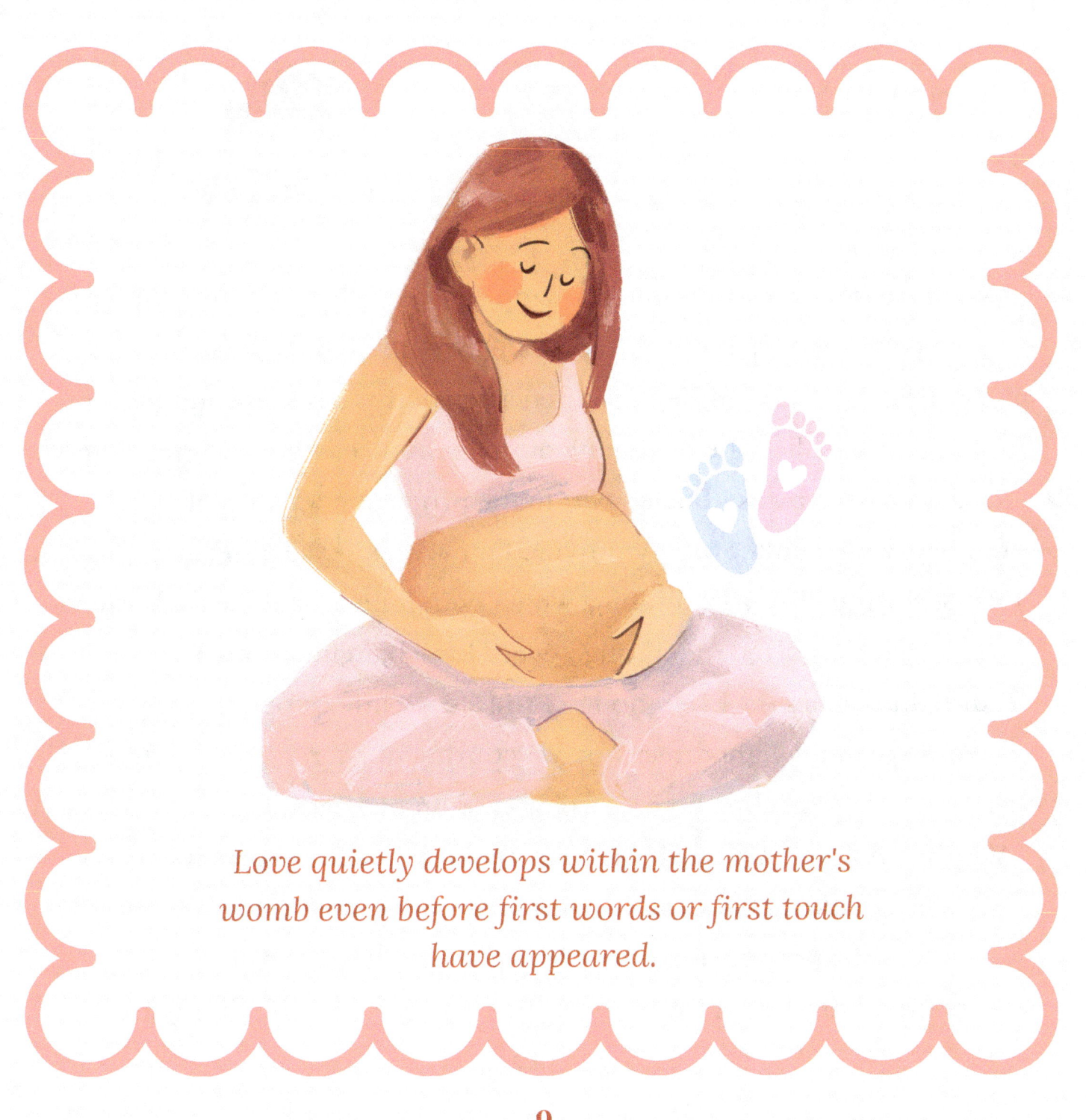

Love quietly develops within the mother's womb even before first words or first touch have appeared.

"Dear Mommy,

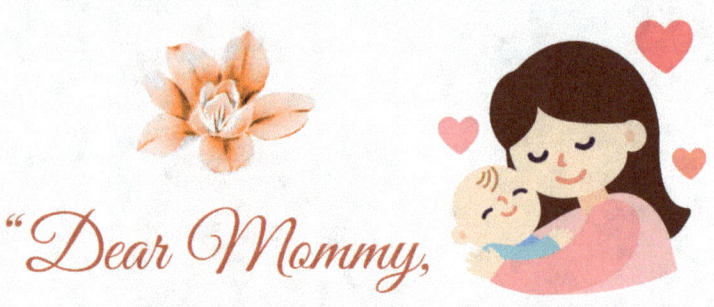

Our story started the instant I took my first place inside your womb as your heart shared its life-creating rhythm and its dreams.

Every heartbeat of your heart formed a protective circle around my tiny body that signalled the beginning of my existence in eternal love. The days passed by as I floated within the protective warmth of your embrace, which unknowingly provided me with a sense of security. Your love performed like a sweet song, which both lulled me to peaceful sleep and supported me through every life-changing moment.

Your light reaches me even though I still sleep without opening my eyes. Your gleaming light directs my way during our serene times while leading both of us forward on our path.

Your womb's serenity enables me to hear the quiet whispers that carry your gentle melodies along with your gentle laughter as well as unexpressed hopes that reside deeply in your heart.

A thousand tiny kisses from my mother reach me as you fill my being with peace.

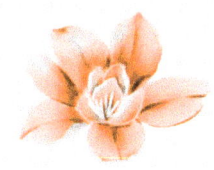

My tiny kicks flutter in the womb as a way to touch your soul by tapping rhythmically to express that I can sense your presence.

I love you.

I'm already yours.

The day I am held in your arms will bring to life the safest experience I have ever known, despite the fact that these moments have not arrived yet.

Each new day strengthens our connection more and more by weaving our love from every single one of your aspirations, your gentle spirit, and your silent courage.

You remain my permanent home while being the initial discovery of my life along with becoming my eternal illumination.

Your love holds me deep within its private refuge, where I clearly perceive that

I am cherished beyond words. I am never alone.

At this very moment I already occupy your heart."

Chapter Transition

"The growth of your power leads me to discover a stunning new beauty which emerges from our connection. Through the process we become something greater than one individual— an extraordinary symphonic composition of two hearts that find musical unity."

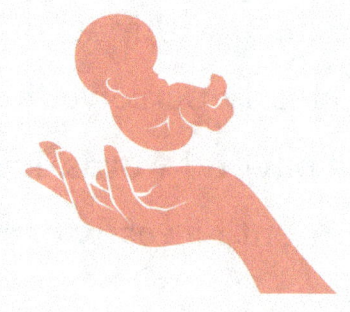

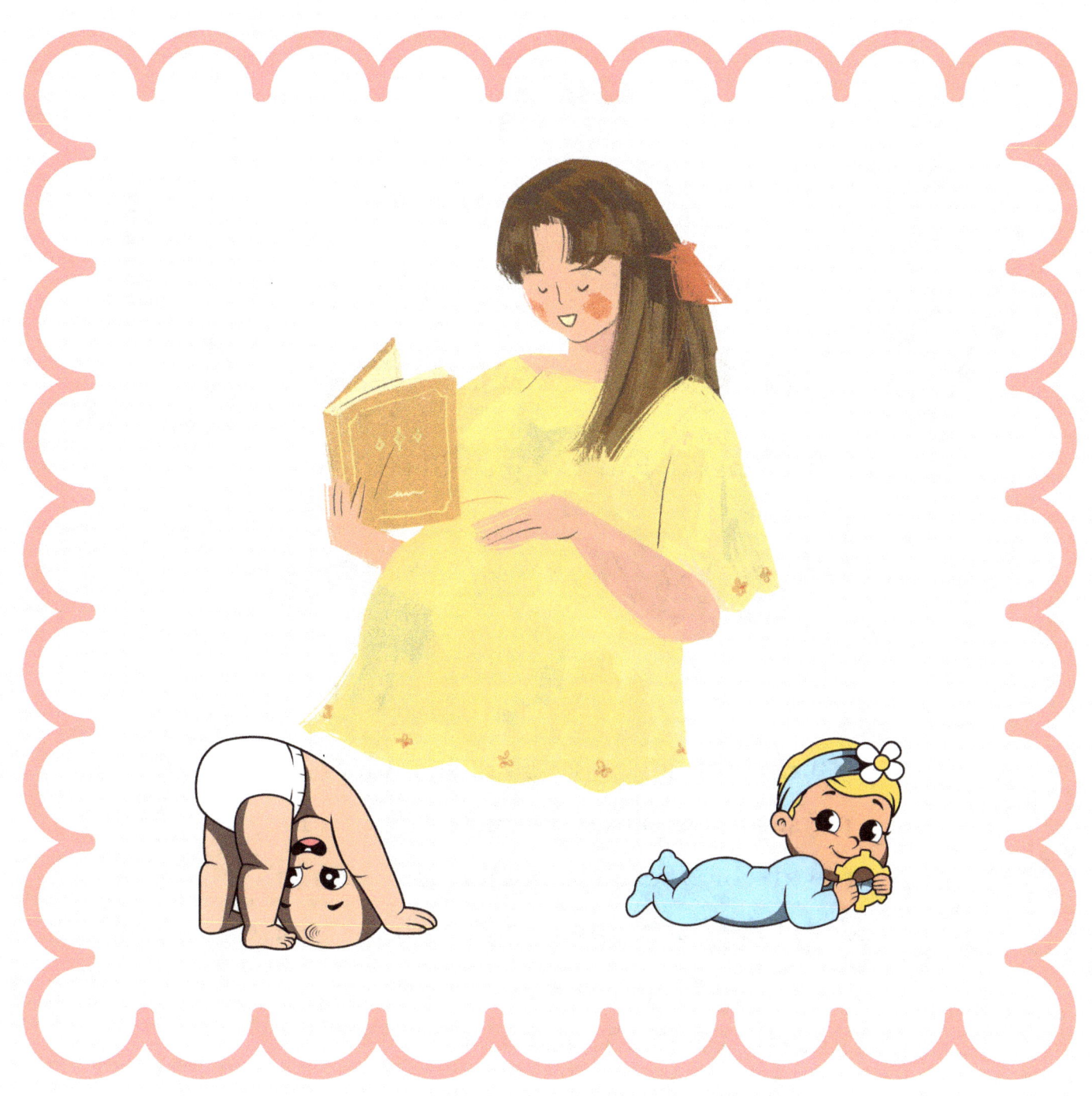

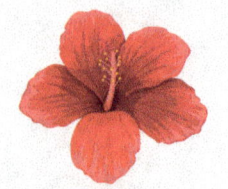

Chapter 2
Growing Together, Stronger Each Day

A shared journey of strength

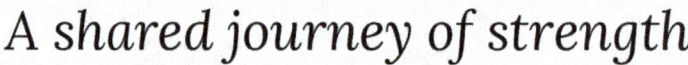

Whispers from Your Baby

"During this journey you have undergone physical as well as emotional and spiritual growth which resulted in increased strength. Look at the unobtrusive ways both of us have been growing to become better versions of our past selves."

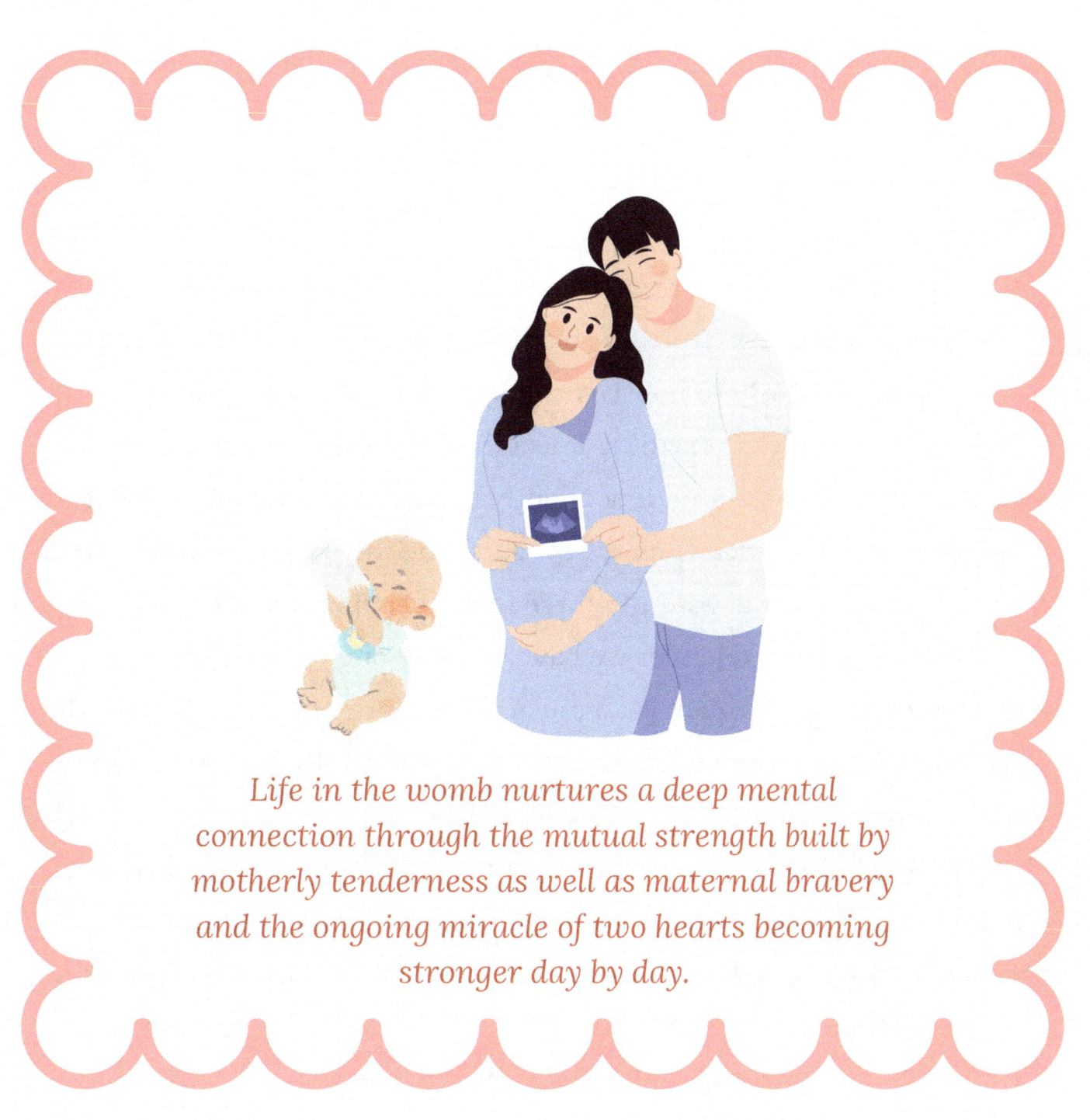

Life in the womb nurtures a deep mental connection through the mutual strength built by motherly tenderness as well as maternal bravery and the ongoing miracle of two hearts becoming stronger day by day.

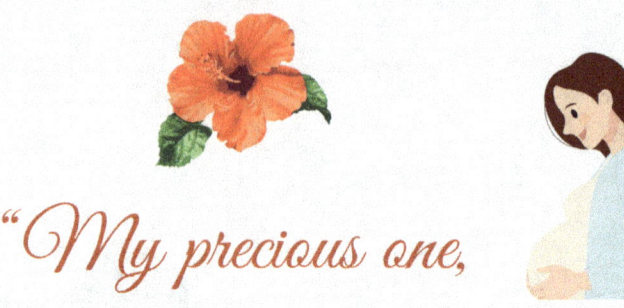

"My precious one,

I develop inside the regular flow of your physical structure. The strength in every heartbeat from your body finds its way into my heart similarly to how rivers enrich a developing ocean.

Your love provides everything I need to thrive while simultaneously showing me how to stand independently before I can even use my legs to tread the earth. This sacred space reveals to me the wild symphony which is your breathing while your life force maintains its constant movement.

Creating our life together we have become one perfect duet that harmonizes its way through each musical creation. The paths of your day may stretch beyond your footsteps so that you would grow weary but I recognize these times.

Your ability to bear me remains so beautiful that it permanently shapes my inner self. The small triumphs and breaths lead me to understand what genuine strength truly means since it manifests as quiet fortitude rather than exhaustion lessness. Each new day discovers deeper penetration of our roots into the soil.

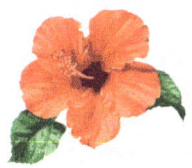

The union deepens in every stretching moment of development when your spirit enhances mine.

Through such an intimate connection we build together, we have forged not just a survival bond but one that grows higher and reaches outward to create a future through measures of courage and softness. Every time you smile while feeling my movements and stop to hold your growing baby, your growing hope draws my attention.

This unexpressed faith drives me forward through my small body and transforms to become the fundamental essence that keeps me alive. You are transforming me at the same time I exist within you. Your strength and ongoing love guide the miracle that becomes the reality of our dreams.

Each instinctive breath you breathe creates irreplaceable promises that meld into our being to become unshakable and brilliant and genuine."

Chapter Transition

"The growth of our strength has brought new changes to the horizon. Transformation approaches and we will welcome it with dignity as a unified group."

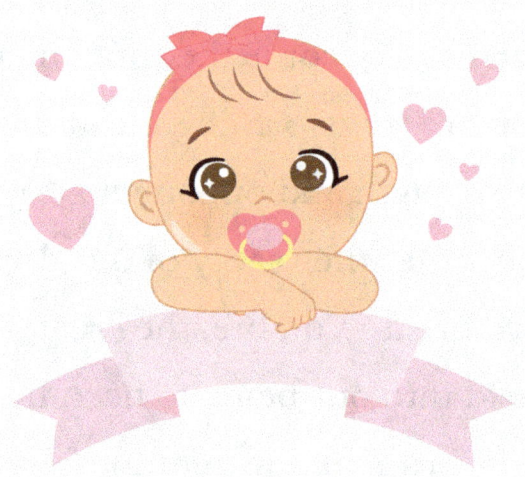

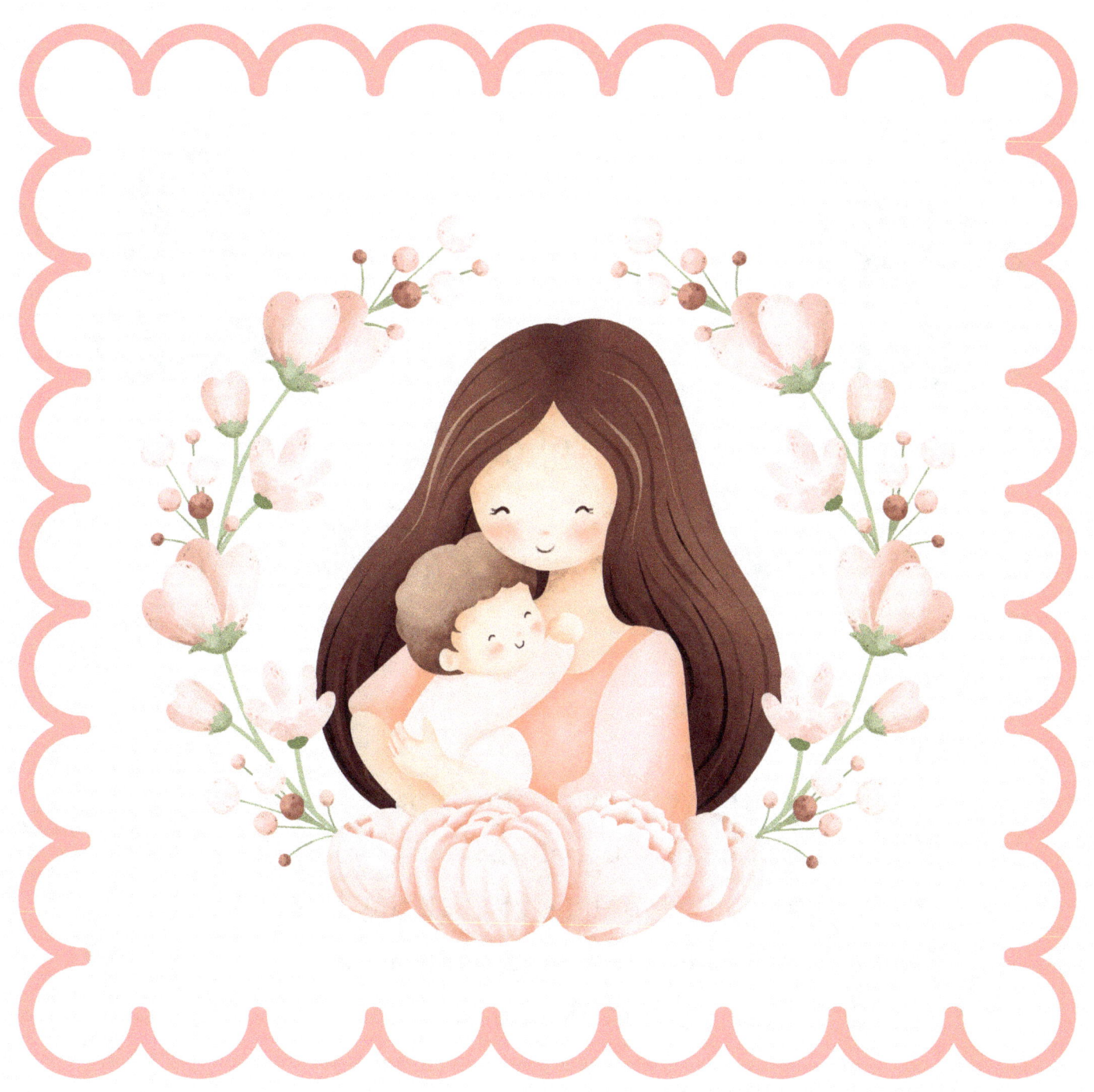

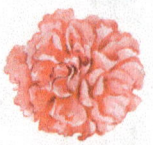

Chapter 3
Nurturing Love, Nurturing Life

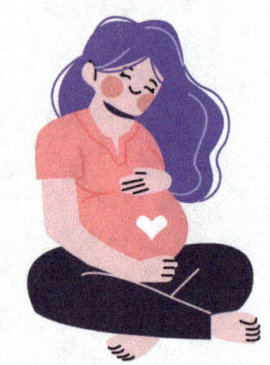

The power of gentle care

Whispers from Your Baby

"Which everyday practices enable you to take care of your baby as well as yourself. Remember to show yourself tiny acts of kindness as your tenderness spreads onto me."

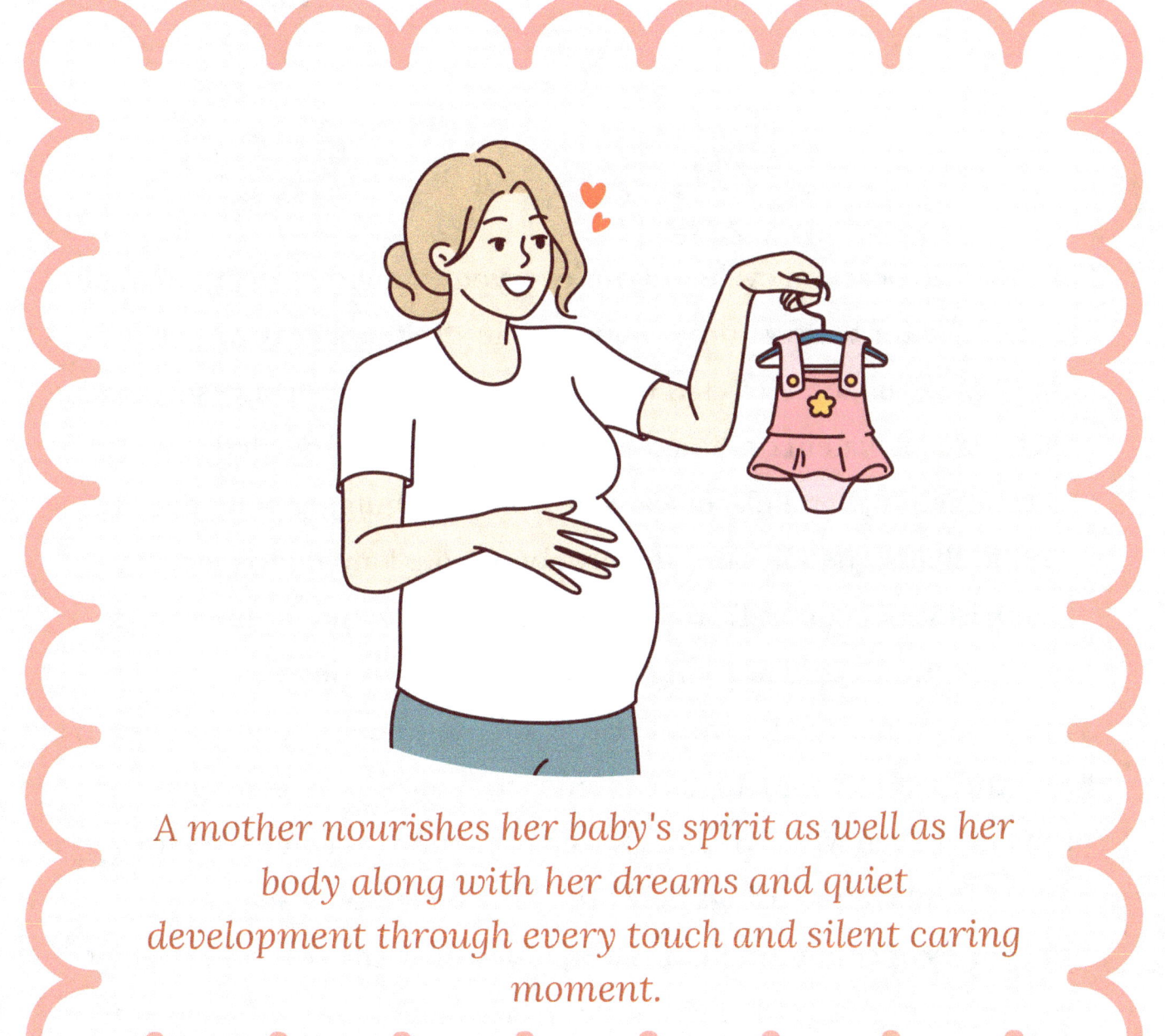

A mother nourishes her baby's spirit as well as her body along with her dreams and quiet development through every touch and silent caring moment.

"My Beloved one,

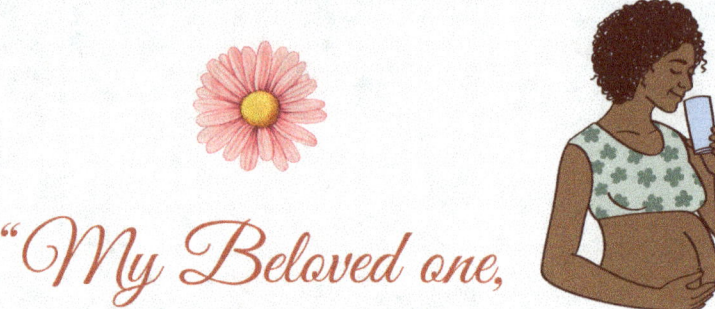

Through the peaceful cycle of your everyday activities I learned about giving love for the first time. Your smallest selflessly caring gestures both for yourself and directed towards me create the strongest impact. Each glass of water combined with every period of needed rest and every touching hand placed carefully on your bulging belly declares aloud that someone cares deeply about you. I am cherished. My nourishment comes from both your offerings and your endless compassionate giving manner that shows devotion.

Your heart functions above all else to keep me alive yet also serves to bring me peace. Your laughter extends to me with the gentleness of a soft blanket even when you laugh solo to the moving wind. Your every inhalation brings new life to my developing self.

Categories of contentment or hopefulness become soft breezes that direct my progress with grace while strengthening me into a person of confidence. The dreams you envision for me float through our surrounding space in an unseen path towards the sun.

Your spiritual love allows me to blossom unnoticed but completely recognized by you. Your spiritual being supports me even though I remain blind to the world before I open my eyes.

Your care creates a musical harmony which uses your presence rather than words to communicate with me. These feelings confirm I am needed and deserve to stay and belong to this place established by a connection beyond my current comprehensions.

I exist beyond physical development of my limbs and lungs. I am growing faith. To believe in gentle love along with the feelings of ownership while getting limitless sacred gifts that request nothing. Every peaceful self-care period in which you dedicate yourself leads to my development.

We create together a safe place which allows compassion to shine through light while life grows unexpectedly in this dimension. You will feel my first touch with my small hands one day thus I want you to remember these words. Your affection has instructed me about how to extend my reach."

Chapter Transition

"Change will soon come to stretch and shape us both...
Our foundation in this peaceful care garden enables us to face all changes during our life journey."

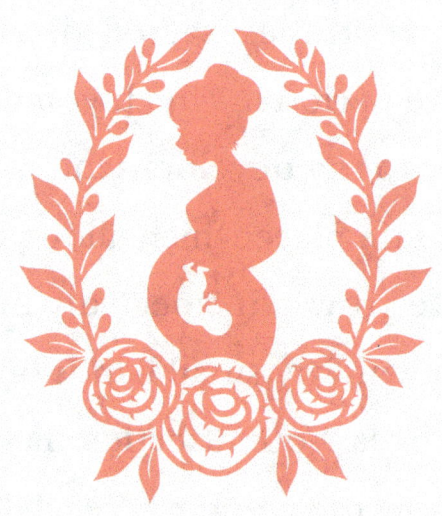

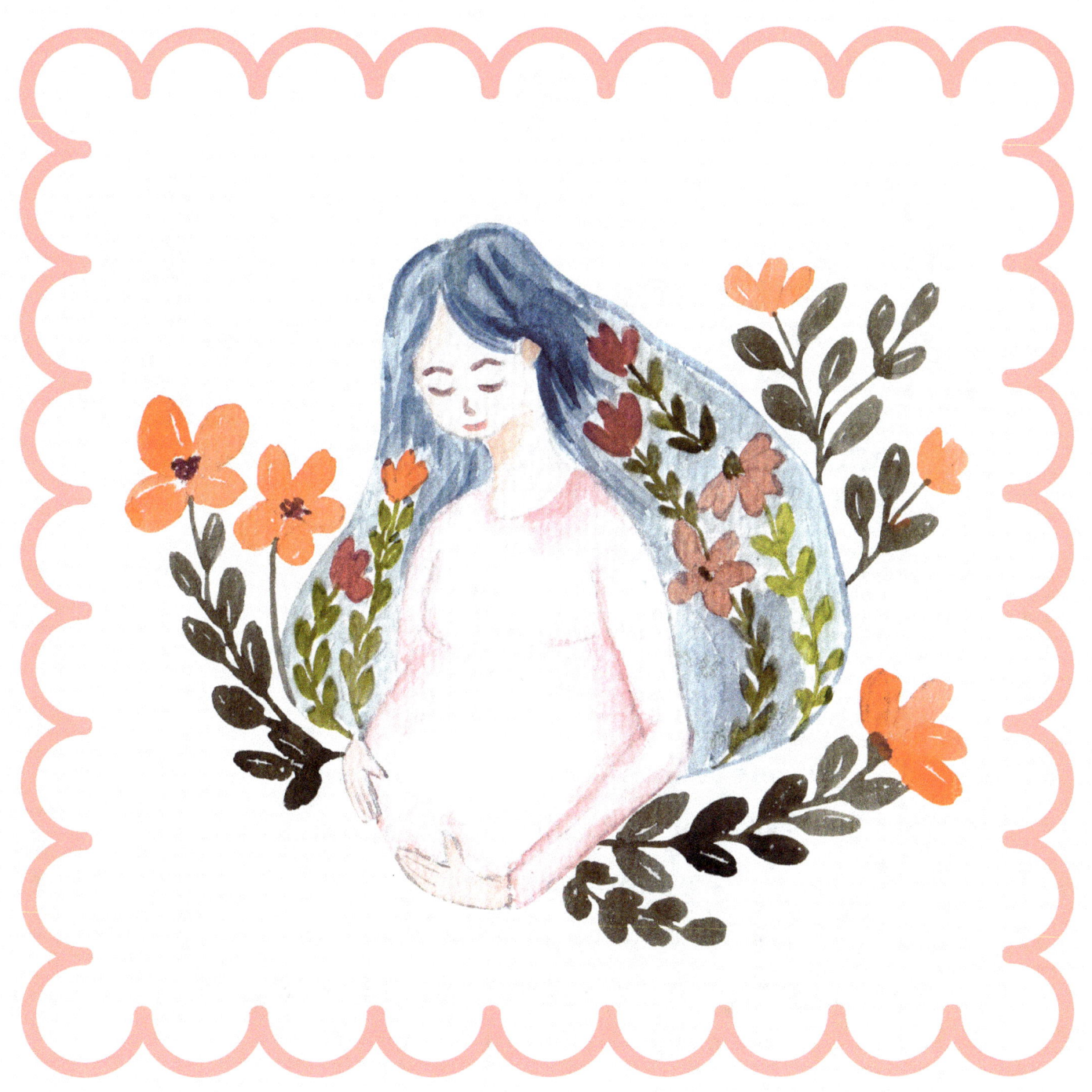

Chapter 4
Journeying Through Changes

Adapting, embracing transformation

Whispers from Your Baby

> "During your trip you adapted differently across physical and emotional and spiritual areas.
> Praise yourself for the adjustments you have welcomed and the tiny actions of braveryyou demonstrate daily."

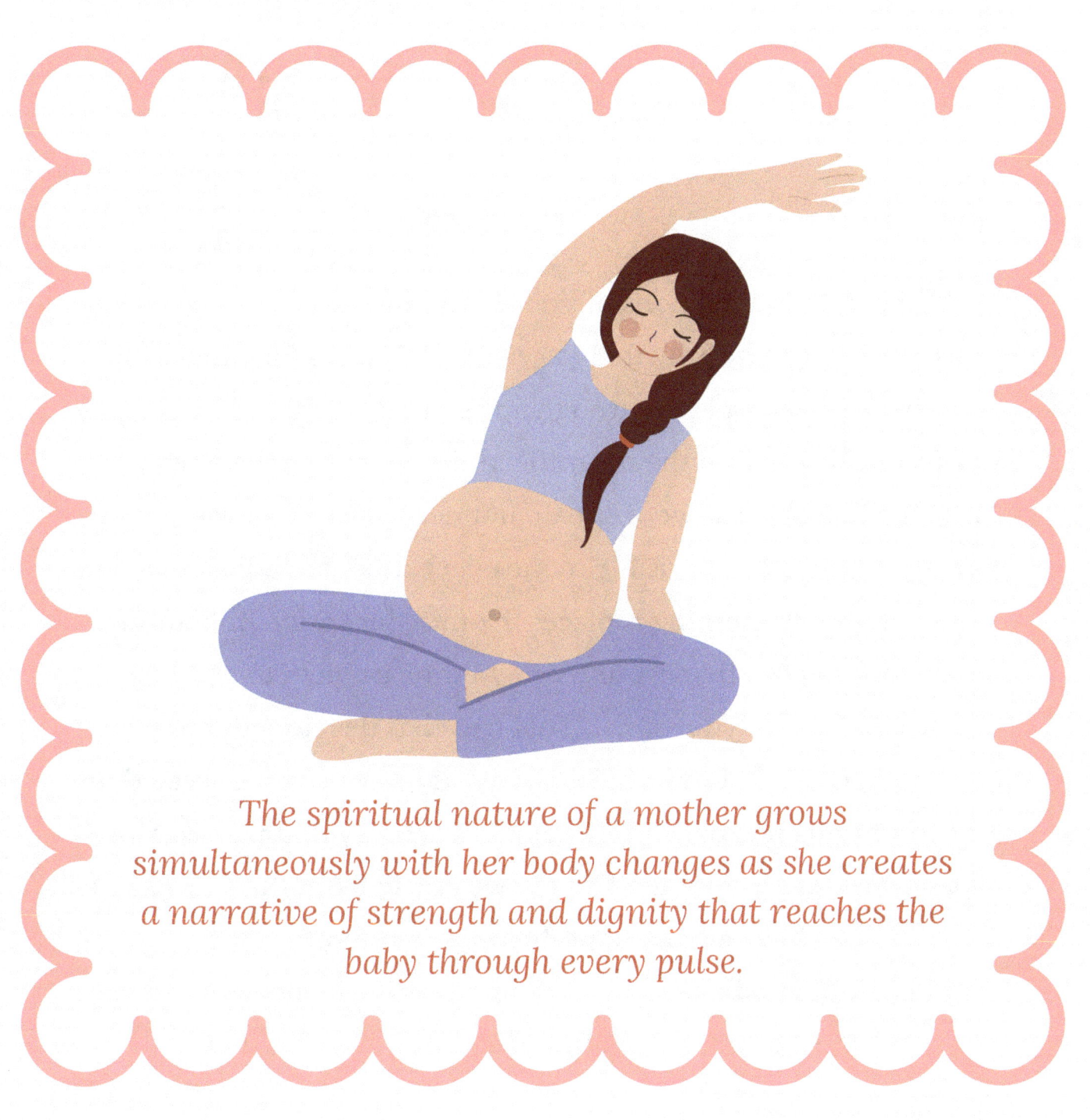

The spiritual nature of a mother grows simultaneously with her body changes as she creates a narrative of strength and dignity that reaches the baby through every pulse.

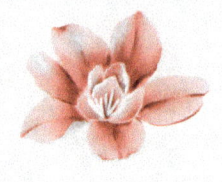 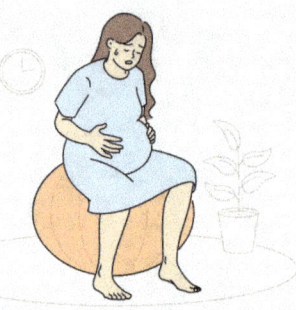

"Dearest heart,

The daily modifications of your body mirror your effort to accommodate my growth. Every physical strain together with doubtful feelings leads us through an astounding dance that shapes our journey to find the magnificent future which lies ahead.

The shifts that occur in your life do not necessarily become simpler. Your strength becomes visible to me every time you adjust to a new phase of life. Blossoming replaces the misconception of bending. The doubts you briefly encounter in your heart yield to a strong and peaceful faith of your spirit. That trust has developed into my bedrock because it shows changes exist as beginnings concealed by uncertainty. You expand your abilities each day that passes. More expansive. More luminous. The life we create from the connection between our souls belongs to us both.

Your developing skin along with your changing heart demonstrates to me that transformation happens through belief.

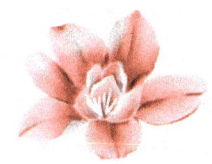

This development of becoming new represents powerful strength rather than weakness.

Your boldness shows through your laughter when unexpected movements happen in your body.

The way you popularize your belly during dark moments of life demonstrates your inner strength.

You continue to trust this process even though you cannot predict all the upcoming steps.

Change transforms you beyond endurance into an active dance partner. Your teachings show that changes in life exist as songs instead of storms which require open-armed navigation.

Your way of life rearranges itself to welcome me into existence. Your love envelops me as I move together with you while you expand your world. Our partnership results in the creation of an exceptional transformation."

Chapter Transition

"The journey through each life change becomes brighter thanks to many small group celebrations which mark both triumphs and sacred moments that hint at upcoming wonders."

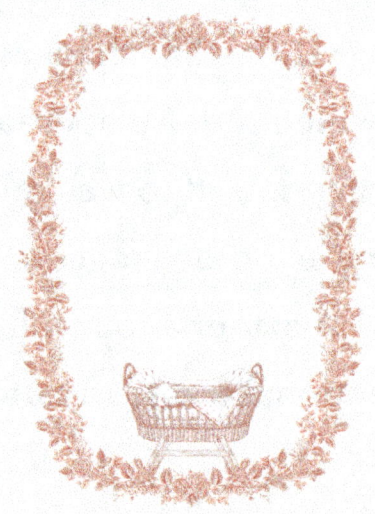

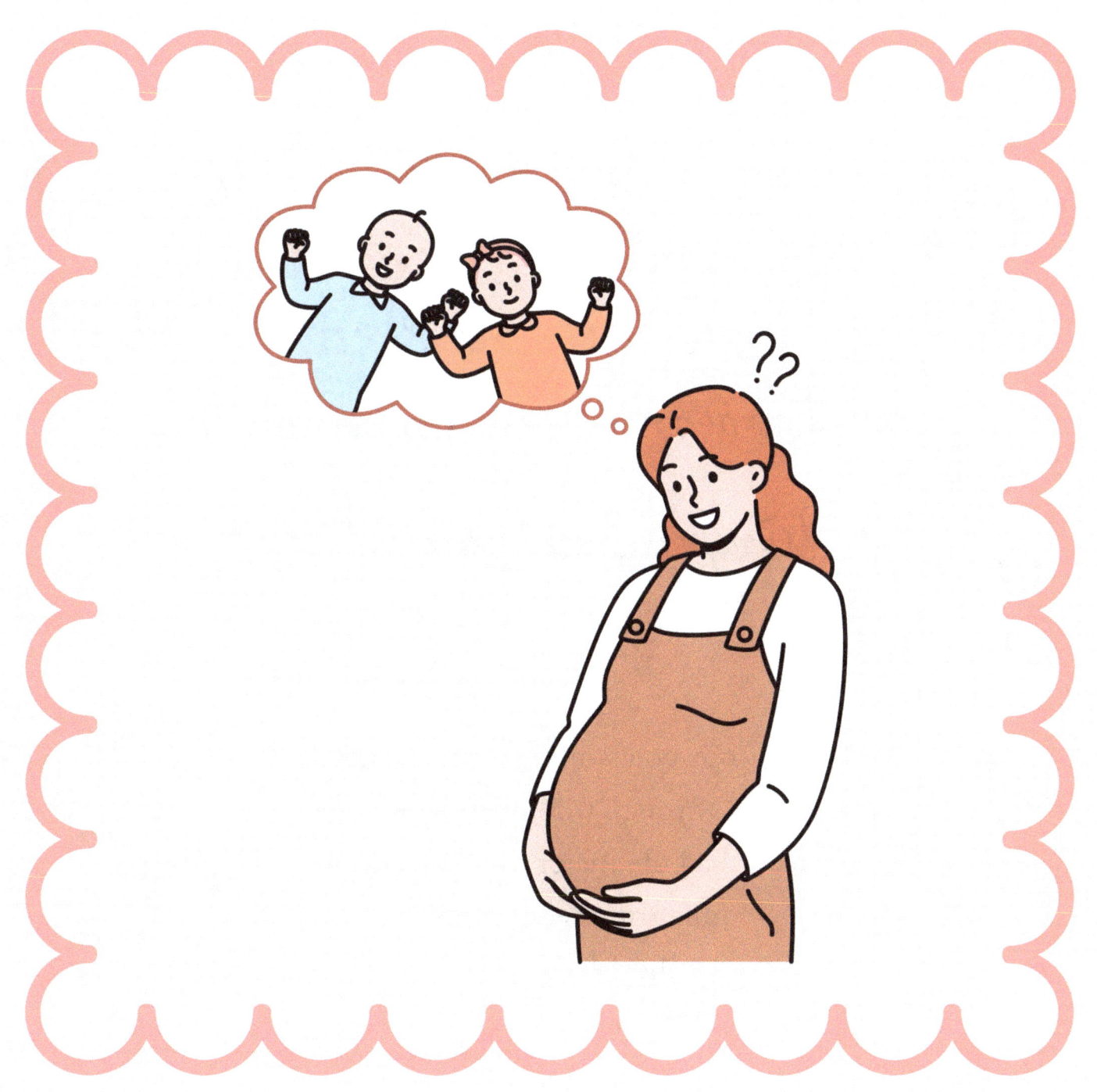

Chapter 5
Celebrating Milestones, Cherishing Moments

The journey is not only about growth

Whispers from Your Baby

"What stops you smiling during your path through this journey?
Record all the major as well as minor milestones you want to cherish forever."

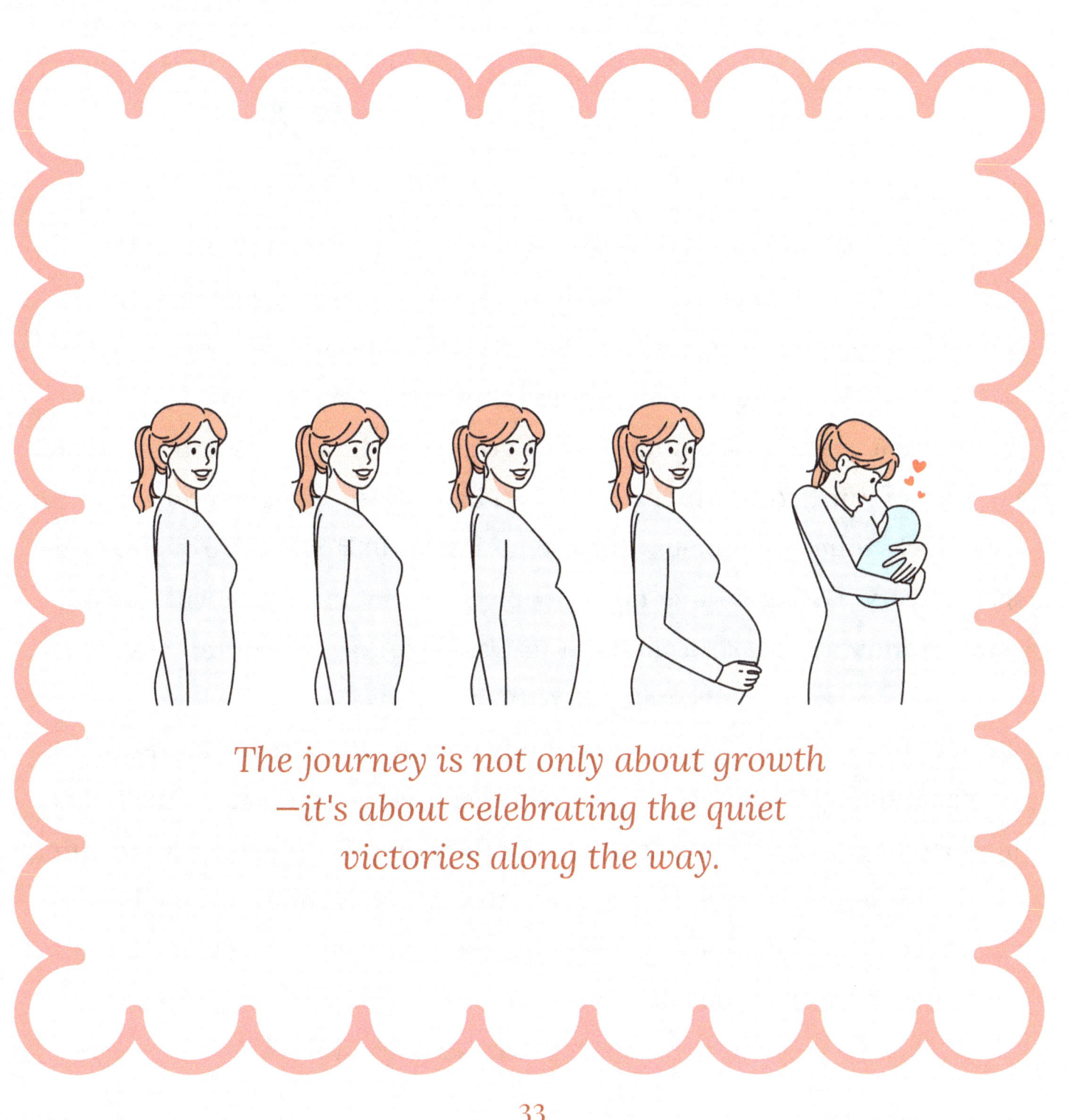

The journey is not only about growth
—it's about celebrating the quiet
victories along the way.

"Sweetest soul,

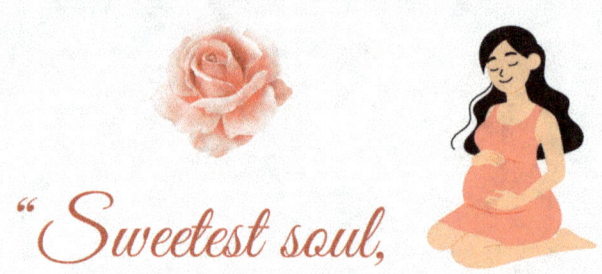

During such moments time seems to stop altogether in the presence of others. We each experience small moments of private achievement which seem to possess our own enchanting secret even though others cannot fully understand them in the same way.

I share that exact same emotion when your heart hiccups after hearing the first beat of mine. You respond with both hands seeking your stomach as my quiet kicks touch your belly which sends beautiful laughter throughout the space. Every passing moment that people share with us along with the quiet conversation we speak through the air transforms into beautiful beads that decorate the path of our lives.

I celebrate every movement of my body because these stretches represent my expanding presence in this world. New movements create a small dance of appreciation which forms a peaceful celebration for the miracles forming within us both. Throughout my life with you you have shown me how to celebrate everyday moments of happiness. Your words to me are always gentle and soft as you talk. Your inner serenity shows itself when you envision everything that lies ahead for us.

Your resting breath establishes a harmonious pattern along with the sound of your voice when you speak and the quality of your inner admiration for the future shines like tiny lights from the string connecting us. Each heartbeat of my whole body expresses joy at watching us accomplish our shared accomplishments. Each accomplishment feels insignificant for others yet our universe considers them magnificent. Your ways of being make me aware of your view which celebrates me for myself rather than my actions and holds me dear. Our dance leads us inexorably toward our first meeting because every important moment including wiggles and heartbeats and smiles urges us toward this face-to-face encounter. The memories from this journey currently reside inside our identity structure. The gentle hands of love have woven shining threads while adding laugh-inducing threads and threads of wonder into existence.

Each passing moment brings to your pure joy that extends to me. Our silent vow affirms we confront each upcoming experience jointly through embracing each other with loving hearts and joyful faces that value the entire time we spend together."

Chapter Transition

"And even in the quiet spaces between
our celebrations, there is beauty—
A peaceful connection develops
between us which transforms joy into
internal stillness leading to power."

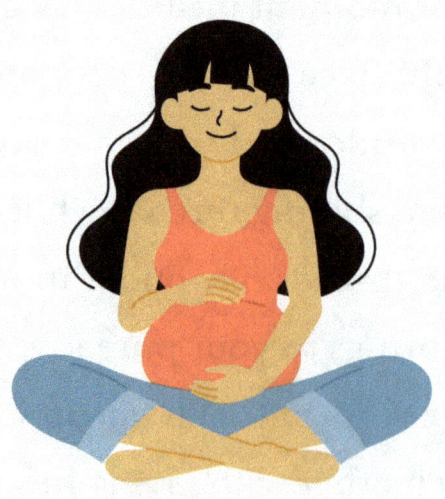

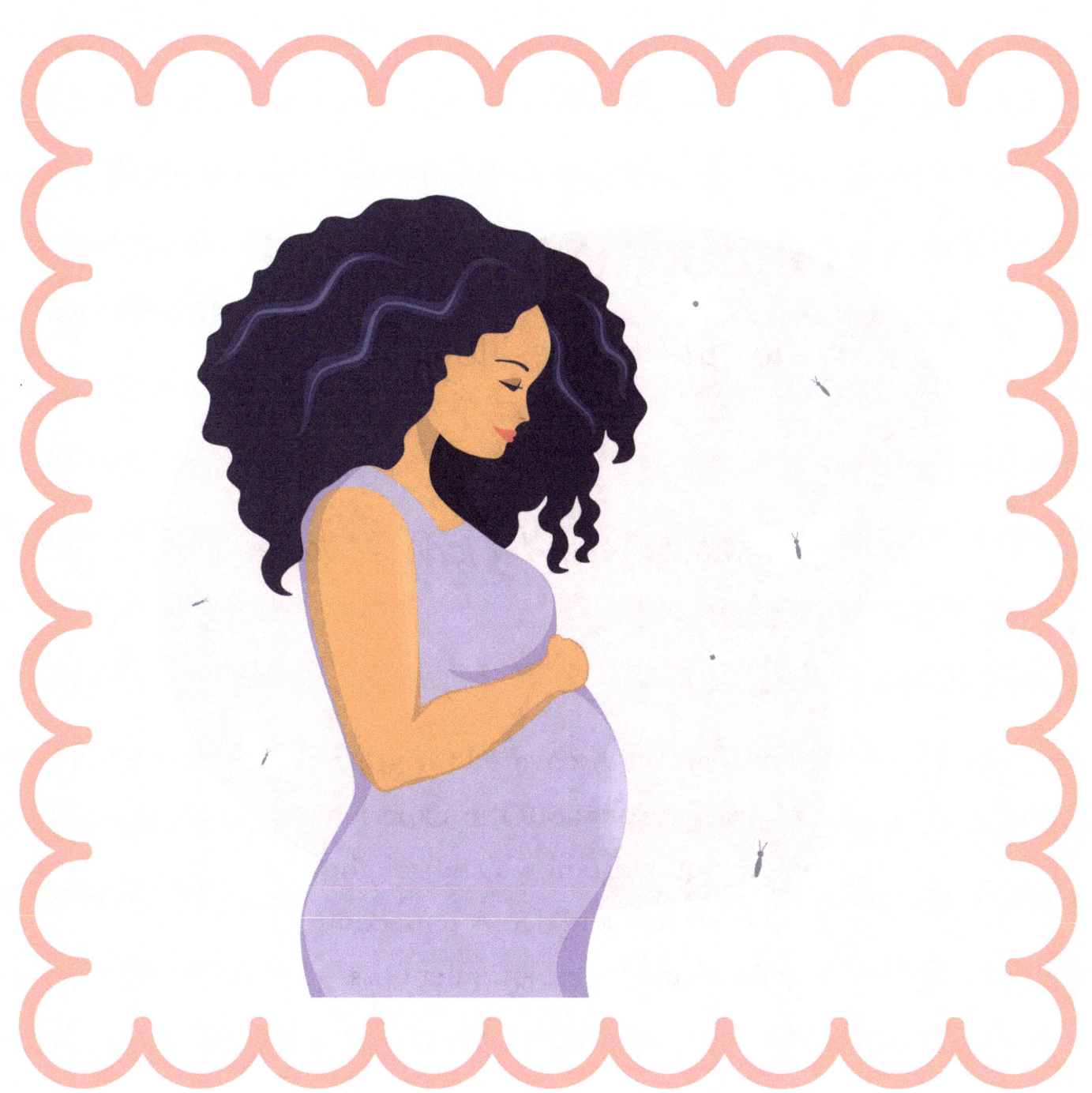

Chapter 6
Finding Peace Within

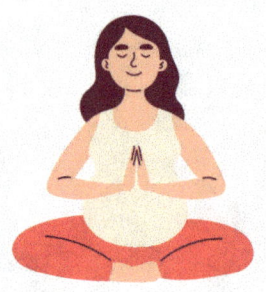

In the quiet spaces, love deepens

Whispers from Your Baby

"When have you discovered the greatest sense of peace throughout this experience? Find one tranquil instant which brought you complete safety and deep connection together with a sense of quiet bliss."

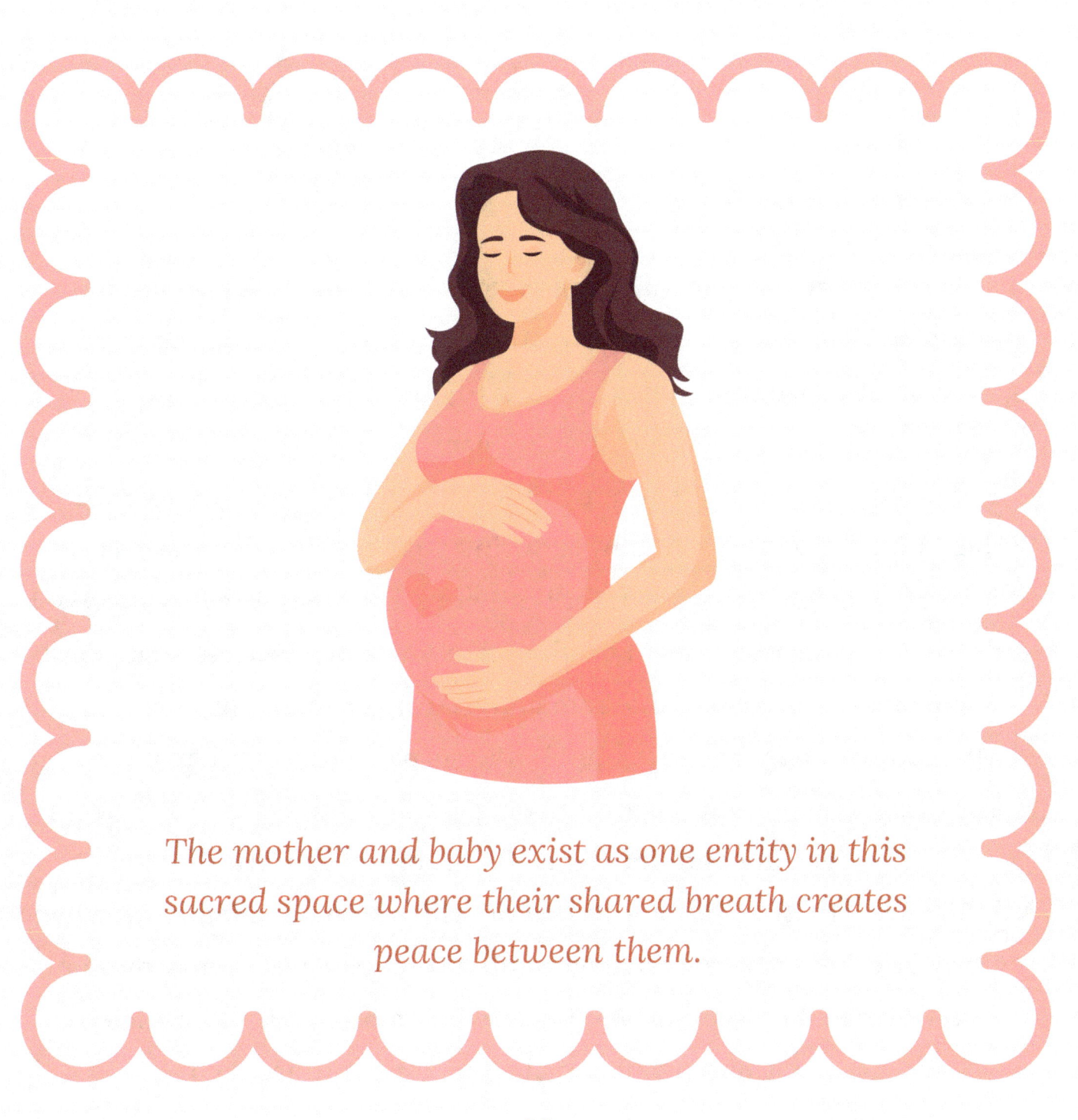

The mother and baby exist as one entity in this sacred space where their shared breath creates peace between them.

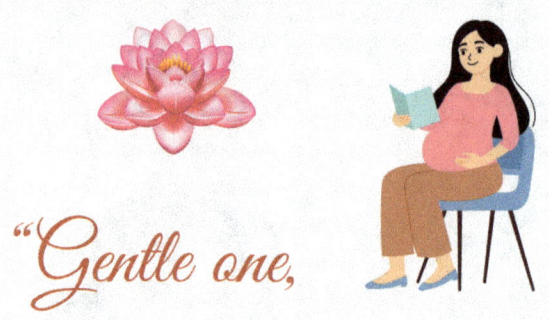

"Gentle one,

I seek refuge in the peaceful space of your heart whenever you remain motionless. The calm pauses between the stress of life bring me to your gentle spirit which tranquilly comforts my heart from your untethered position in place.

The essence that appears when you remain silent turns into my most cherished music. Deep breathing during your eye closures makes the entire world seem to slow down for both of us. The deep breaths allow our souls to intertwine more deeply with each other. Your peaceful state exists deeper than oceans while remaining stronger than any storm.

Entry flows to me through channels that surpass any verbal expression. Home exists as an emotion because being cradled, understood and deeply loved unconditionally is what represents home.

A divine peaceful state resides inside you which remains silent even when outer world noises fill the environment. A serene peaceful environment exists where I find both protection and belonging with my sufficient existence while joy plays its mystic tune.

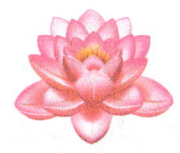

The soft promise of your hand placement on my body always brings out this unique sensation to me. Your prayers to the stars reach me silently. My spirit drifts upon it as you give your body permission to rest because you trust complete nourishment exists inside us. Your peaceful demeanor educates me about how to develop trust for the very first time.

You show me peaceful methods to breathe and dream and hope beyond angst when you remain calm. The construction of my physical being is only part of your profound influence because you serve as the lifeboat shield to my soul.

When my eyes finally open to view the world I will carry with me the calmness which existed all along. Life will take us to places but your peaceful presence understands that tranquility exists at every location where you reside.

Thank you for the quiet.

Thank you for the stillness.

I thank you for establishing my first protected sanctuary."

."

Chapter Transition

"When you rest within this peaceful state a radiant light emerges inside you which radiates its warmth beyond me to shine for all the world."

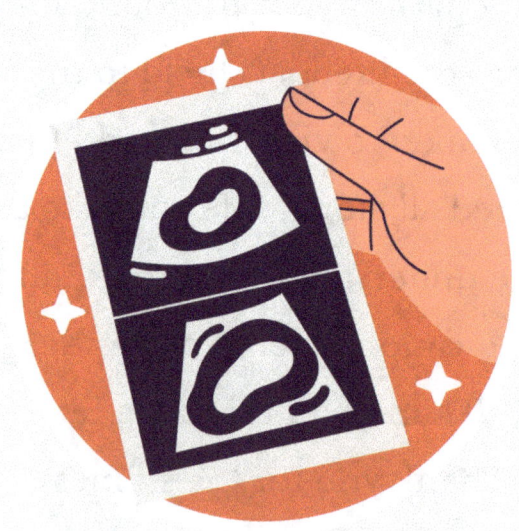

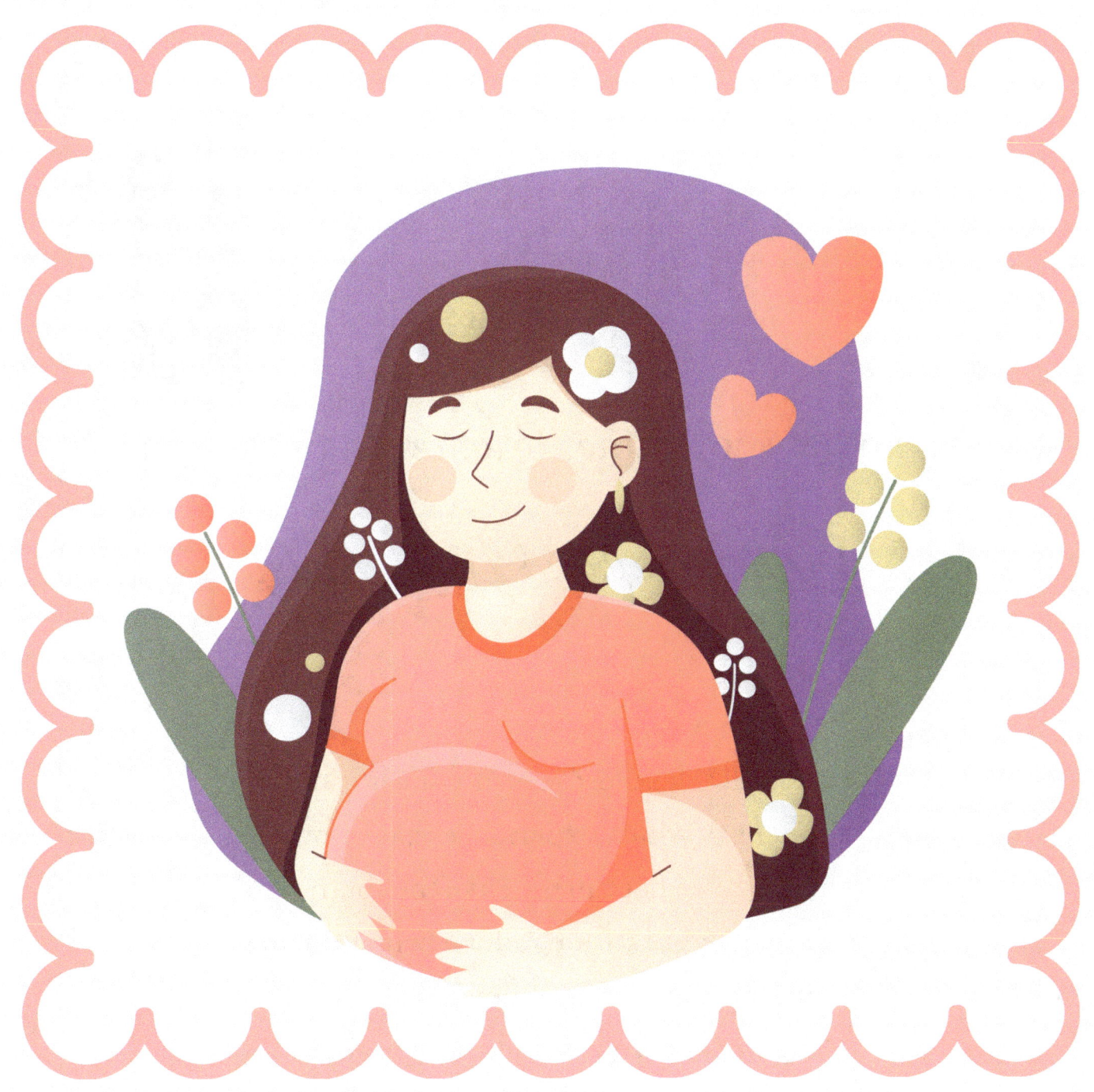

Chapter 7
Radiating Love and Light

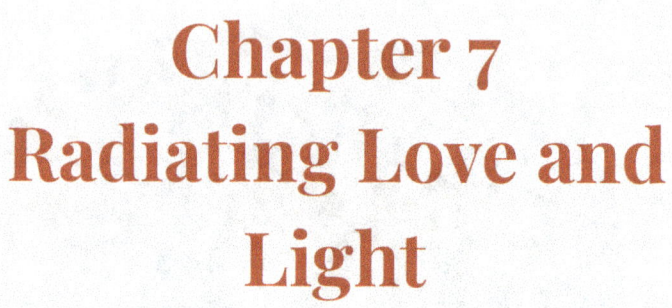

A mother's joy shines brighter than the sun

Whispers from Your Baby

"Recall the milestones of your life and identify which experiences gave you genuine pure happiness. Save the memories that made your inside radiate bright during this journey because they contain your laughter and your pride and your light."

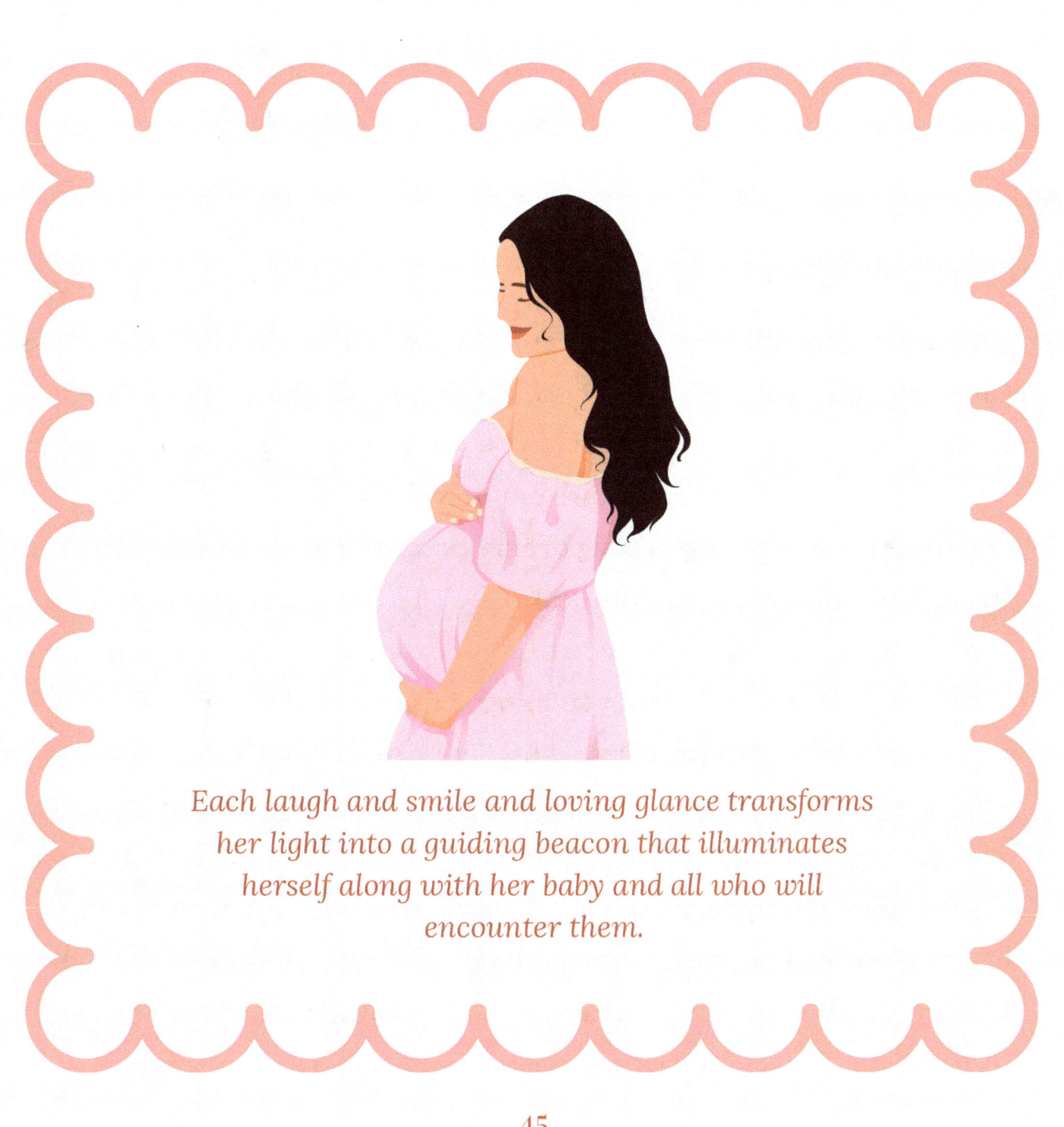

Each laugh and smile and loving glance transforms her light into a guiding beacon that illuminates herself along with her baby and all who will encounter them.

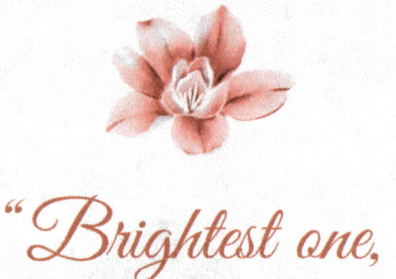 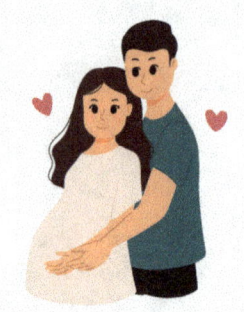

"Brightest one,

I feel your light. The light blankets me completely with dynamic golden tendrils that protect all areas of my personal realm from the chill of shadows. Fear cannot affect the light you possess inside which glows forever bright. Your liveliness appears in the singing you produce during your daydreams about future opportunities.

Your laughter shines with sparkling beauty because it wells up from within to bring us both upward in each musical note. The entire inner cosmos within you alters completely once you express happiness with your smile.

Your light spirit lifts all around you into a tender state that seems to attract even celestial bodies nearer.

Your happiness belongs to both of us since it exists beyond being yours alone. The experience fills my heart with amazement to show that life serves purposes beyond its quiet existence. Surrounding you both with streams of light starts when you whisper words and hold me gently since these light streams pass through your soul and reach my vulnerable heart. The light radiates through my closed eyes so I can perceive its essence.

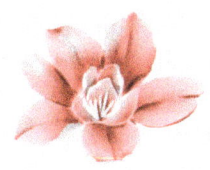

The way you exist in life combines with your affection and natural radiance that shines automatically. You are my first sunrise, My first glimpse of hope, A belief started in me that beauty exists past these peaceful waters.

Your love teaches me that light exists within us rather than being a pursuit. It's something we are. We develop into individual beings when we allow ourselves to encounter happiness during moments of unknown direction.

Thank you for being my light, for laughing with abandon, Your smile retains its strength through all circumstances as it provides comforting feeling and creates warmth and true happiness in people.

Your dreams along with mine shine with a radiance darkness can never diminish because you skillfully carry them forward.

Our upcoming venture will lead us to different locations because the following lesson will accompany us everywhere we travel. You shine such beautiful light that I will always find my way back home to you."

Chapter Transition

"The dance of your light brings nourishment to my spirit while also energizing your own spirit. Through continuous mutual sharing true love generates the energy required for new developments to emerge."

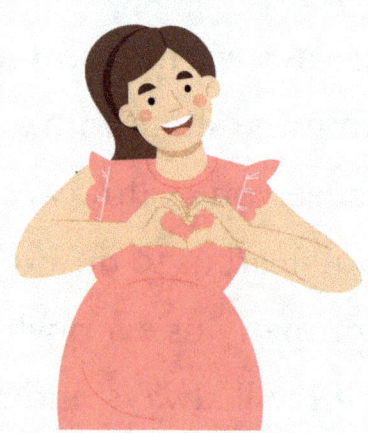

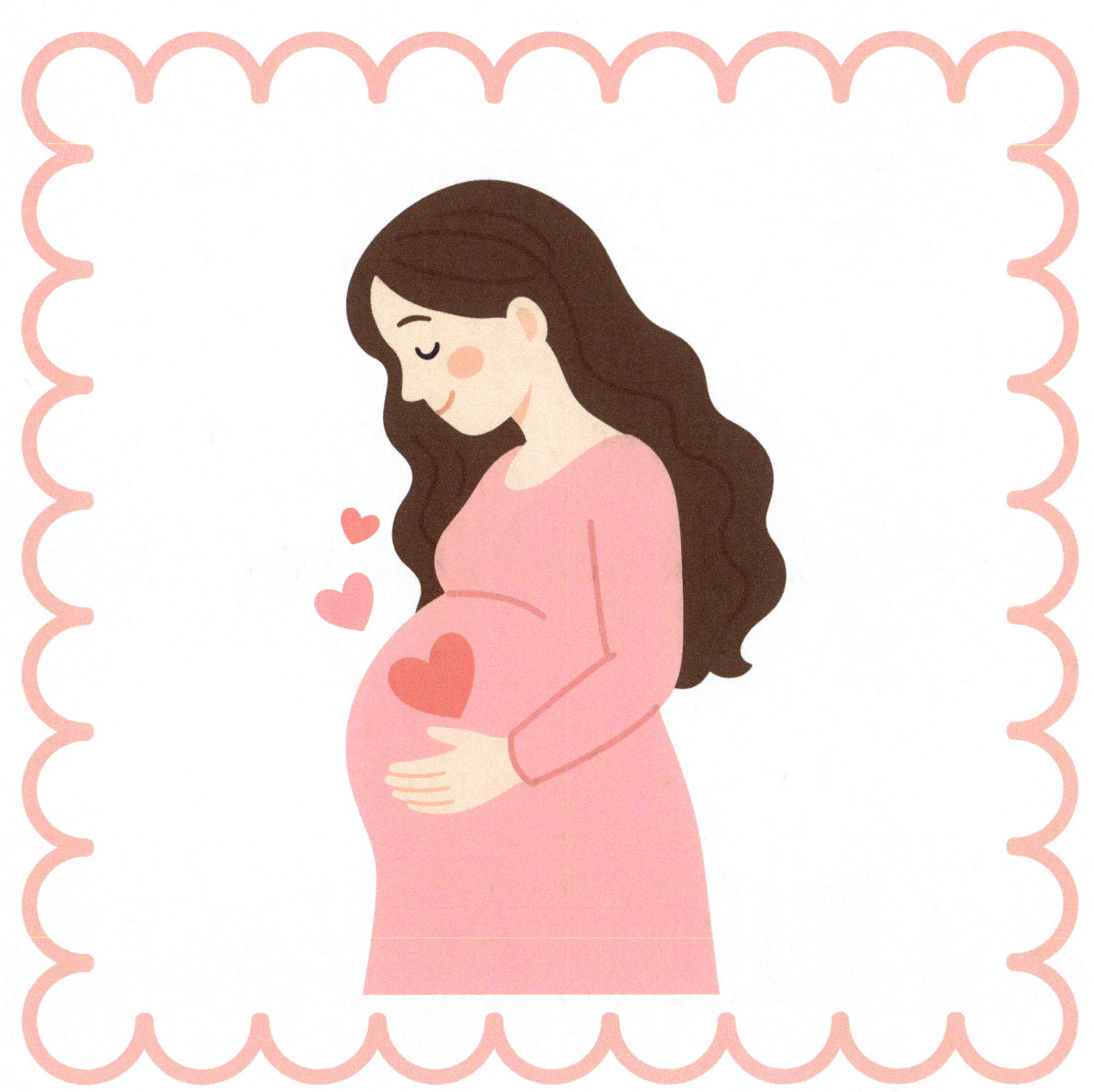

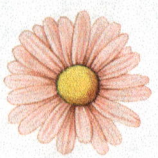
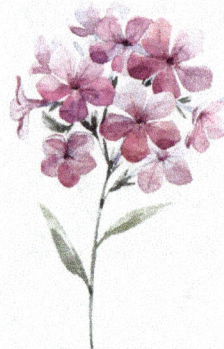
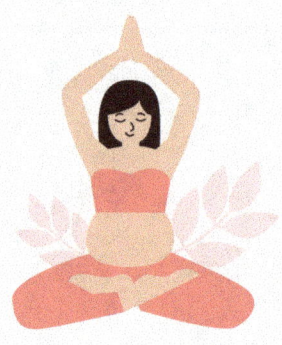

Chapter 8
Nourishing Body and Soul

Every act of care you give yourself nourishes both of us

Whispers from Your Baby

"Modern self-nurturing presents
an important question.
Note down the simple routines that bring
rest or enjoyment or caregiving to help
you value your amazing path forward."

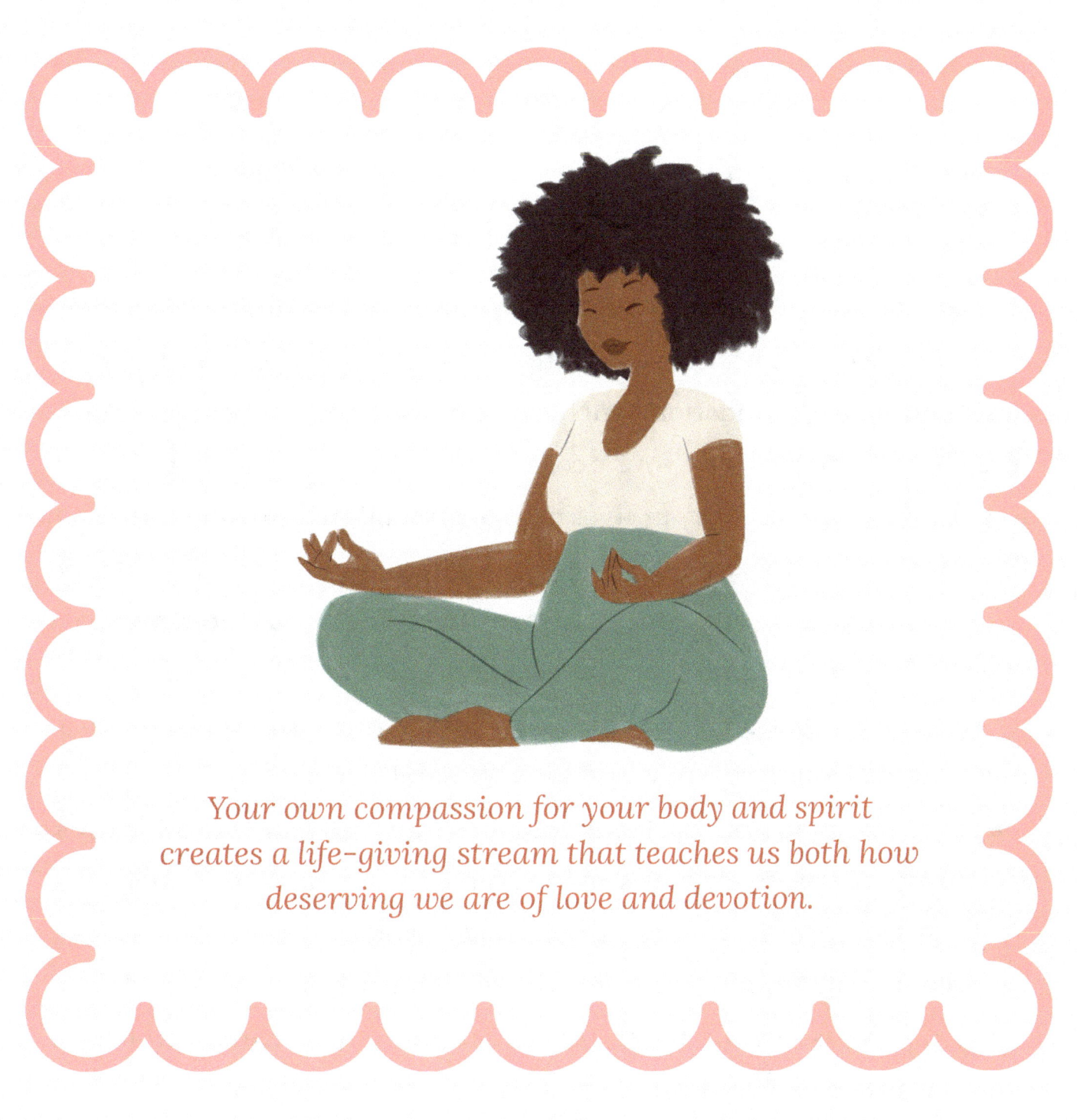

Your own compassion for your body and spirit creates a life-giving stream that teaches us both how deserving we are of love and devotion.

"Beloved heart,

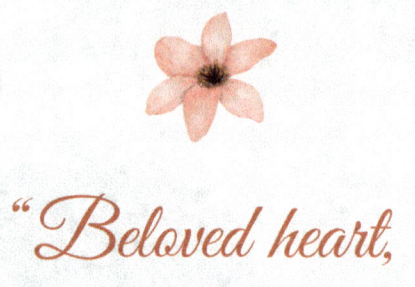

I sense every love you show yourself. Your body's breathing relaxation combined with water consumption and food intake establishes a sustaining life foundation which exists below both our beings. Your practice of taking care of your needs communicates to me that: We are sacred. The worth of both our lives calls for intentional slowing down. The thing we nurture together deserves the highest level of care. Each action that shows your caring appears as sweetness when you prioritize rest instead of urgent behaviour and select gentle attitudes instead of criticism or self-condemnation. You serve as my initial instructor to display that might stems from gentleness and loving oneself emerges from self-care. The act of self-nourishment feeds you both physically and emotionally so it becomes retroactively a blessing I receive from you. A continual quiet acknowledgment flows through our bodies and cells to connect us by forces beyond mere existence. We are connected by devotion. The cooking pleasures and water drinking routine and dream nurturing process in your mind form part of my development.

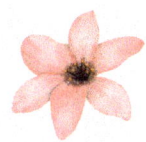

My spirituality develops through the influence of these beneficial elements in the earth. The world's abundant nature lessons me to trust before I have observed it.

A new life grows within you that consists of more than biological matter. Your soul simultaneously develops the awareness of deep love because it knows you are being treasured and supported as a sacred being. Your decision each day to dedicate care toward yourself has built a path of gratitude from my heart.

You selected self-care at each opportunity while it seemed more comfortable to ignore your own needs. Your love continues flowing along each mouthful and throughout each breath and beneficial act you send to yourself although you remain unaware of the positive impact it creates in my life.

I thank you. Your self-care demonstrates to me the fundamental reality which states that you are deserving of love. The worthiness to be loved extends to me because it extends to you."

Chapter Transition

"With love from you, both of us grow stronger while facing an uncertain path ahead which now appears bright. The forthcoming year delivers bravery together with faith and vast opportunities beyond fear."

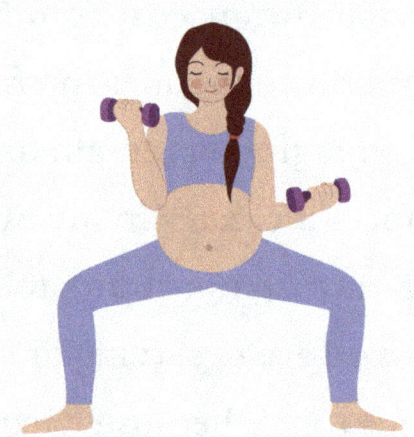

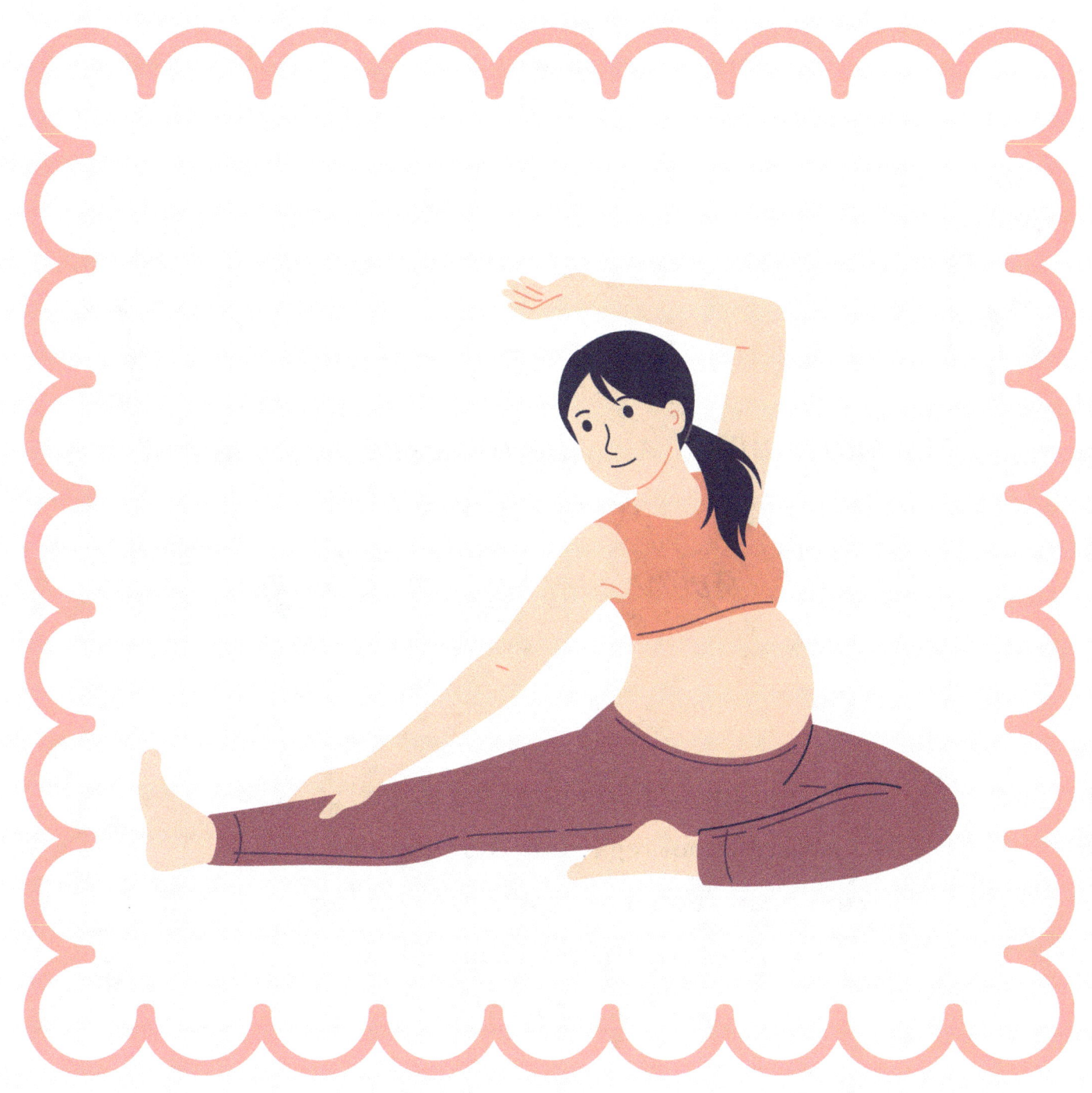

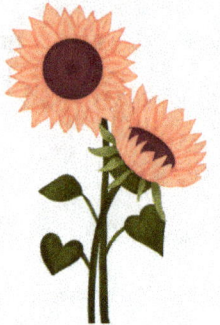

Chapter 9
Embracing the Unknown, Trusting the Journey

The path ahead may be unseen, but it is not traveled alone

Whispers from Your Baby

"What things do you hope for as well as worry about regarding the future? Your heart should discuss the upcoming mysteries and the trust you hold to overcome them."

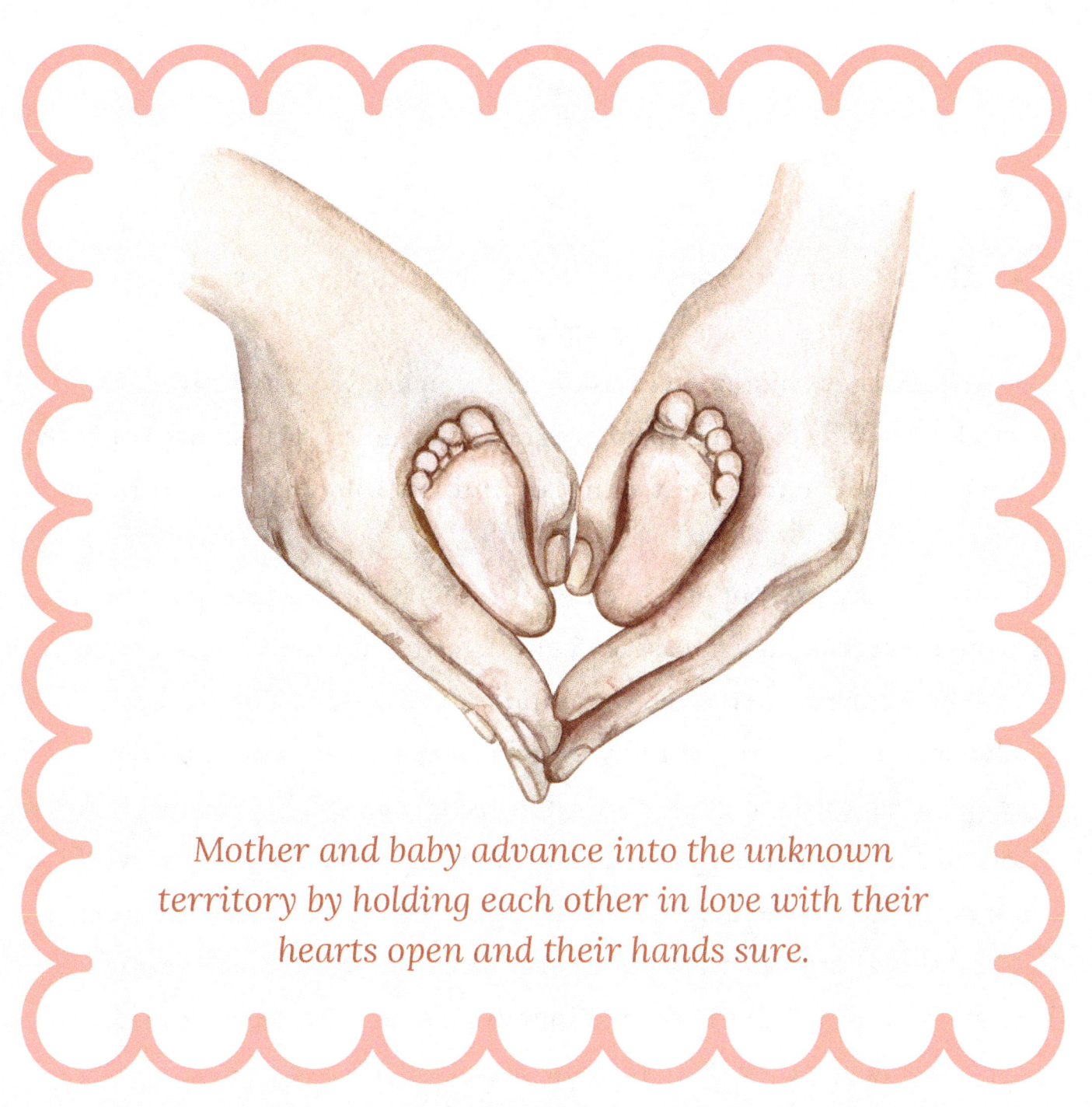

Mother and baby advance into the unknown territory by holding each other in love with their hearts open and their hands sure.

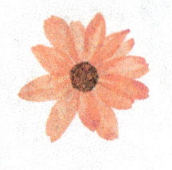

"Bravest one,

The path forward consists of a narrative which we have not yet experienced.

The message is hidden in invisible ink which reveals itself gradually through breathing and heartbeat progressions and small instances of faith. Several times I encounter feelings of limitless wildness in the coming phases of life.

The infinite sky in front of you extends forever until it steals your breath. Through every unknown passage your determination becomes visible in the same manner as ten thousand radiating stars. The road to advancement requires no full view of all steps ahead. You should only depend on the loving force which leads us forward. My dearest you possess a love which surpasses every single fear that exists in the world. Your courageous selection of hope is what I recognize in your demeanor. You show compassion to your heart when the world pushes you to become hardened. Your belief in hidden spiritual miracles arises from the way you trust them to grow silently inside your being.

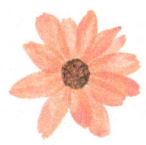

The path leads us ahead with companionship beyond the realm of uncertainty. Future mothers receive strength from all maternal insights that have ever existed.

A timeless love guides our way although our minds have yet to discover it.

The way you teach me shows that unknown situations give birth to new opportunities rather than threatening my existence. An invitation guides us to hope while we believe seeds are emerging from darkness to reach the sunlight.

We should advance toward the future with a strong and fearless spirit. We walk ahead together with our hearts and hands open as we keep a quiet assurance that all discoveries will unite us. During instances when doubt shakes you know that:

I will stay close to your heart while softly reteaching you this first piece of advice.

You are not alone. You never have been.

You never will be."

Chapter Transition

"The future approaches with its gentle sacred vow which brings forth this fundamental truth: Our everlasting love supports us from one start to another becoming to each everlasting stage."

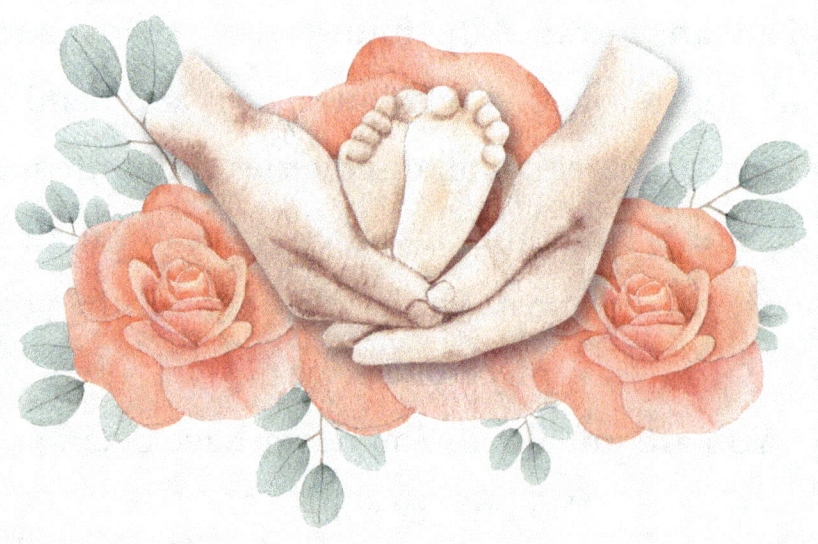

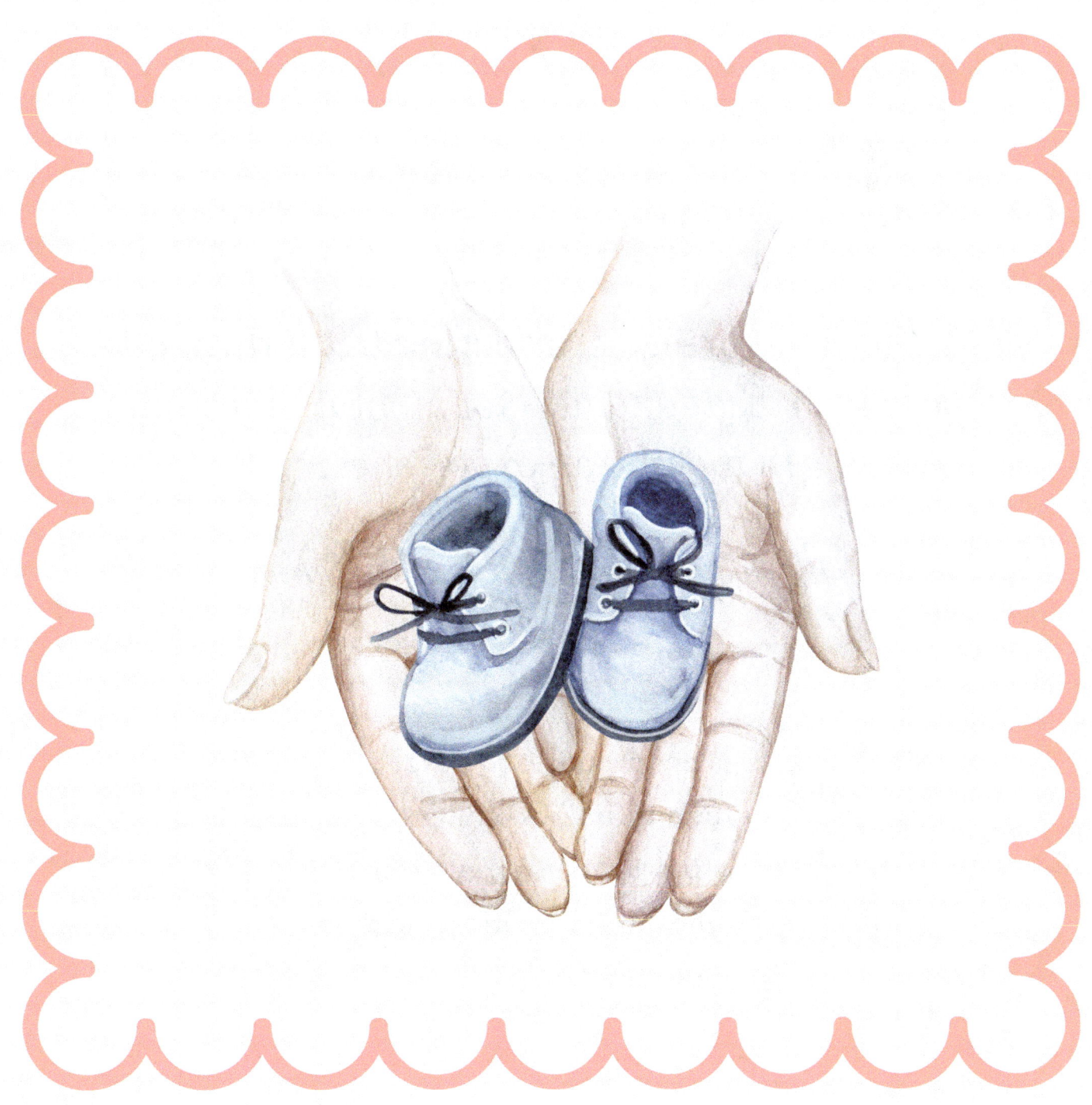

Chapter 10
A Promise of Love

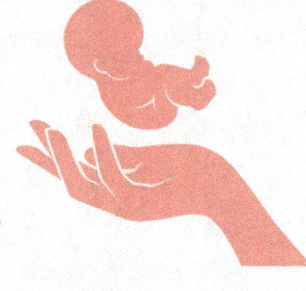

Motherhood brings everlasting truth through every heartbeat and developmental milestone that children experience.

Whispers from Your Baby

"You keep silent promises to me as you wait for our first encounter.
Every vow and dream dear to your heart that will define our future life should be captured now."

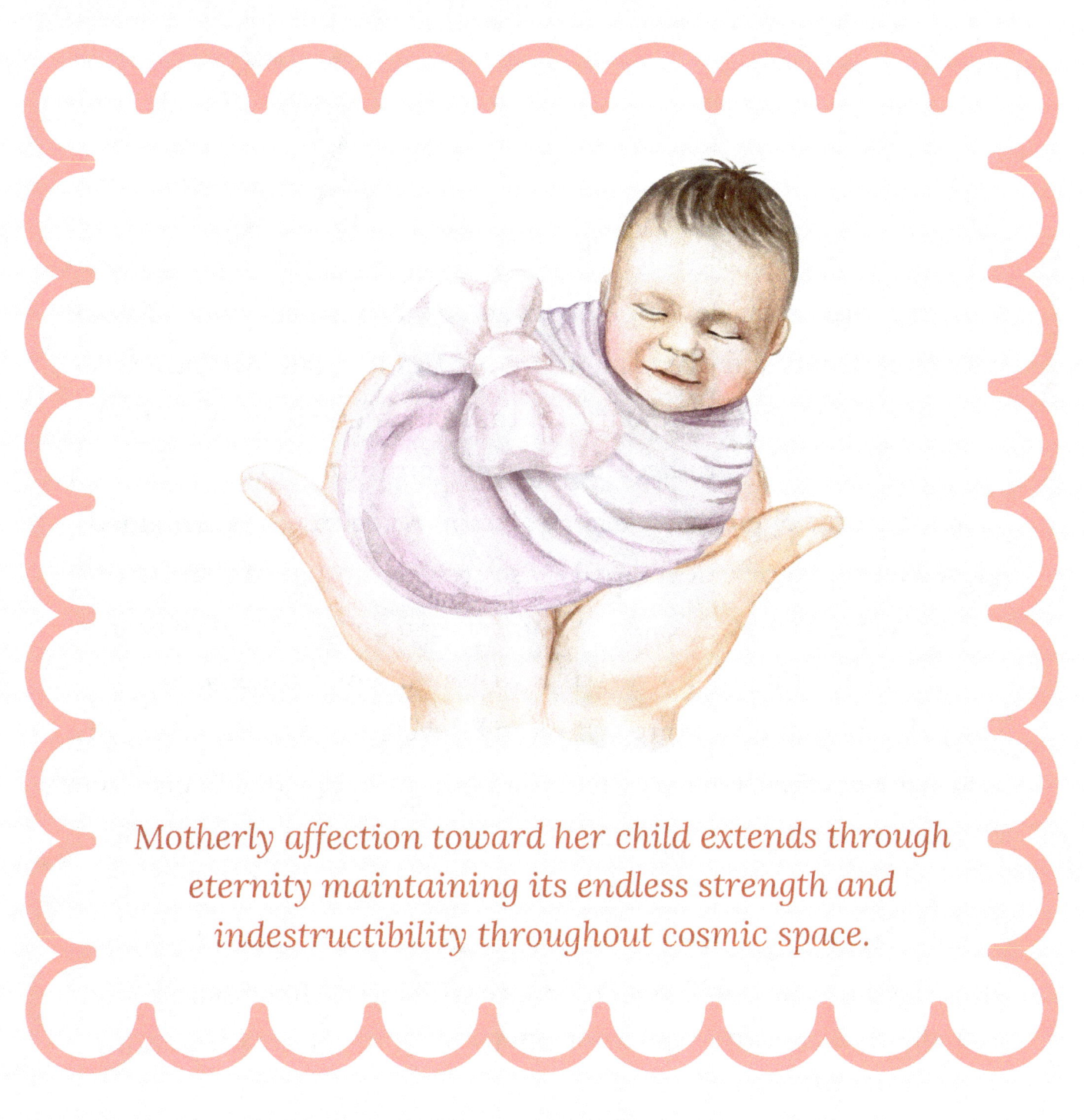

Motherly affection toward her child extends through eternity maintaining its endless strength and indestructibility throughout cosmic space.

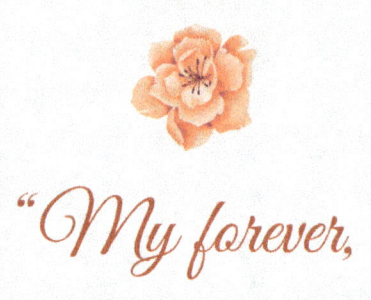
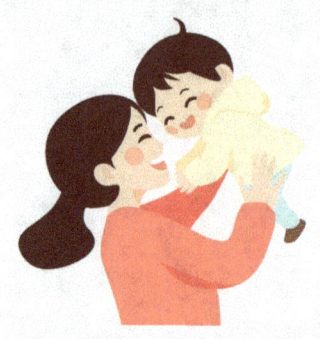

"My forever,

A silent promise has developed between us during every one of your secret heartbeats and every silent breath. In silent faith we know that genuine love has no boundaries because it emerged from genuine intuition rather than spoken commitments.

Your message of eternity began its lesson when my eyes remained closed and my voice developed no song yet you started sharing the language of everlasting love. Your love can be heard within each heartbeat you possess. It is written in your dreams.

The principles of it run throughout my developing identity. This life holds whatever path may come my way because I pledge to keep our bond forever. I promise your love will provide the foundation for my existence as roots in the earth.

From the heavens above I will extend down to the ground so that they become one. I will keep the place which feels like home inside my being forever. All of my life I will recall your unwavering courage whenever I encounter obstacles.

The elevation of my spirit will reveal your joyful laughter that ascends with my flight.

When life becomes vast and untamed your embrace will function as my guiding light to return home. Your light which I have received will remain with me forever.

The light you provided me will become the shining centerpiece throughout my entire existence. I will pursue the dreams you developed for both of us until their completion.

The new aspirations I create will blend with your original love story through its golden essence. Time and distance along with all transformations will never defrost the bond which we created through these silent days.

You are my beginning. You are my guide. You are my forever.

I carry your love within me throughout all time since my first day of existence. I will carry your love in me - glowing, living, eternal.

This, I promise you. "

Concluding Message for you my love

""Dear Mommy,

At the moment of writing my last message to you I feel what our love has expanded since our first meeting. Our upcoming partnership will be filled entirely with the love and gratitude which flows from my heart to yours.

You safeguard me without fail while being both my shelter and all that matters most to me. Through your heartbeat I found my peaceful sleep and your voice brought emotional contentment while your love provided me direction. From my earliest days within your womb until now I have recognized the comforting feelings which came from the way you hugged me.

From today until our lives' end, I will stand beside you sharing happiness and extending support when needed and giving you my wholehearted dedication.

You held me tenderly during pregnancy and spent your life nurturing me while holding an endless love for us both. The treasure of our bond will never cease to exist.

You are the one I belong to forever.

With all the love in my tiny heart,
-Your little one."

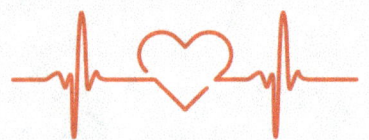

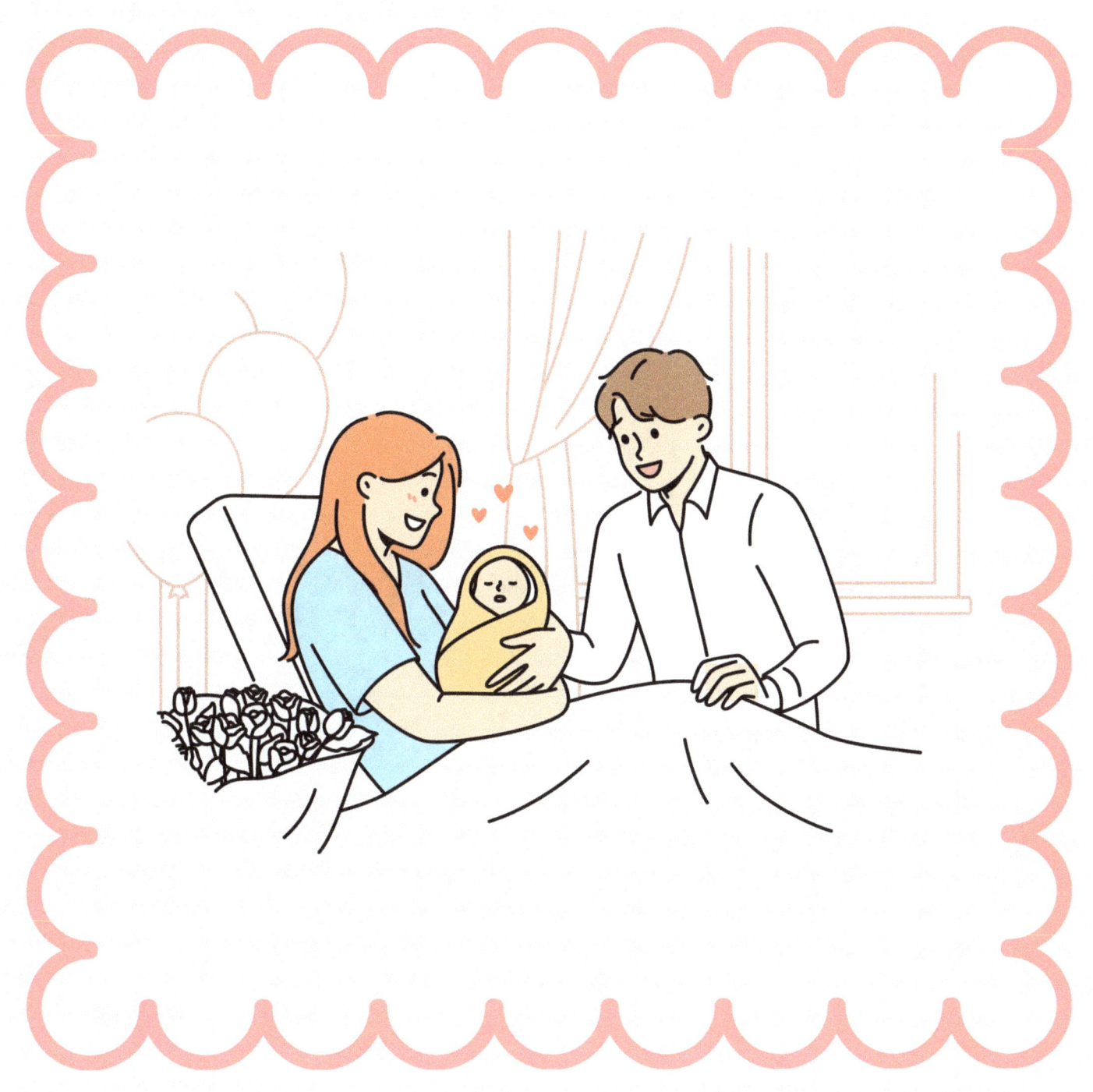

Note from the Author

"Dear Mama,

Thank you for giving the whispers entrance to your heart. I express my deep gratitude.

May your life pathway carry abundance of love together with its illumination and become stronger through your relationship with your child.

Thank you for allowing these whispers to touch your heart. May your journey continue to bloom with love, light, and the unbreakable bond between you and your little one.

Wishing you
Happy Whispers of Warmth!!
Keep Loving! Keep Smiling!"

With all my heart,
Vicky V. Choudhary

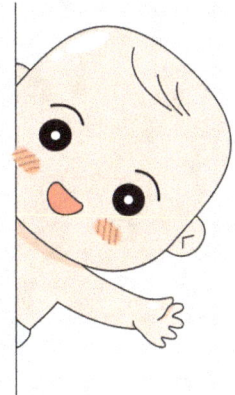

www.ingramcontent.com/pod-product-compliance
Lightning Source LLC
LaVergne TN
LVHW061948070526
838199LV00060B/4023